The Obesity Remedy cookbook:

Recipes to Help You Lose Weight quickly, Manage Insulin, and Improve Your Health.

By

Mason E. Hall

Table Of Contents

First Off

A major global health concern that now affects millions of individuals globally is obesity. Poor eating habits are one of the main causes of obesity, which emphasizes how crucial it is to develop healthy eating habits in order to avoid and control obesity. This book seeks to explore the reasons why encouraging nutritious eating habits is essential to the fight against obesity and the advancement of general health.

Understanding Obesity: Obesity is a multifaceted illness marked by excessive body fat accumulation, which often arises from an imbalance in energy expenditure relative to energy intake. The main causes of this imbalance are sedentary lifestyles and poor eating habits. Promoting healthy eating habits is a key component of any holistic strategy to address the obesity epidemic.

Poor Eating Practices' Effect on Obesity

Obesity and weight gain are caused by unhealthy eating practices, which include consuming processed and sugary meals in excess, high-calorie snacks, and portion sizes that are too large. Over time, weight gain results from these habits because they cause an excess of calories that the body stores as fat.

The Function of Nutrient-Dense Foods: Developing healthy eating habits requires giving top priority to foods high in nutrients, which are foods that are high in vitamins, minerals, and other vital elements but low in calories. Fruits, vegetables, whole grains, lean meats, and healthy fats are some examples of these foods. Foods high in nutrients not only improve general health and feed the body, but they also lower the risk of obesity.

Portion Control and Mindful Eating: Creating healthy eating habits requires both learning to regulate portion sizes and engaging in mindful eating. People may better determine their level of fullness by eating slowly and paying attention to their hunger signals, which can help them avoid overindulging and control their weight.

Regular Meal Routines: Creating a regular meal schedule will assist in controlling blood sugar levels and lessen the chance of unhealthy food impulsive snacking. Regular meal timing encourages a more balanced nutritional intake and reduces the risk of abrupt energy surges and collapses.

The Function of Water Intake: Healthful eating practices include both the meals and drinks that are eaten. Throughout the day, sipping enough water will help regulate hunger, keep you well hydrated, and lessen your chance of ingesting high-calorie or sugary drinks.

Taking Care of Emotional Eating: Emotional eating may lead to weight gain since it entails eating in reaction to stress, boredom, or other emotions. Reducing the need to resort to food for consolation may be achieved by learning more constructive coping strategies for handling emotions.

The Influence of Social and Environmental Factors: Managing and preventing obesity requires fostering an atmosphere that encourages a healthy diet. Encouraging wholesome food options in communities, businesses, and educational institutions may have a beneficial impact on people's dietary choices.

Long-Term Health Benefits: Children and adolescents may lay the groundwork for lifetime health and well-being by adopting healthy eating habits at a young age. Early obesity prevention lowers the risk of several chronic illnesses, including heart disease, type 2 diabetes, and certain malignancies.

Sustainable Weight Management: Rather than turning to drastic measures or crash diets, sustainable weight management emphasizes slow, consistent development. Developing appropriate eating practices is crucial to reaching and maintaining a healthy weight throughout time.

Working together with medical experts: Medical professionals are essential in helping people adopt healthy eating habits. Experts such as registered dietitians and nutritionists may provide customized nutritional guidance and assistance based on each person's requirements and objectives.

Educating the Public: It's critical to spread knowledge about the role that healthy eating practices have in managing and preventing obesity. Public health campaigns and educational programs may provide people with the information and resources they need to make wise food decisions.

In summary, healthy eating practices are the cornerstone of successful interventions for managing and preventing obesity. A proactive approach to improved health and weight management may be taken by people by focusing on nutrient-dense meals, portion control, and mindful eating. Creating conditions that are encouraging and getting competent advice also increases the chances of long-term success. When combined, these initiatives have the potential to help people and society alike have a healthier, happier, and obesity-free future.

Checklist for Healthy Weights

With the daily barrage of media stories about obesity, weight, and health, people may feel overloaded. Nonetheless, there are simple things you can do to control your weight and lower your risk of acquiring several chronic illnesses.

The Healthy Weight Checklist is a useful tool for anybody working to maintain people's health, including parents, caregivers, educators, healthcare professionals, workplace coordinators, public health practitioners, business and community leaders, and healthcare policymakers.

Eat a balanced diet.
Calories are crucial for weight reduction, and some foods improve our ability to control how many calories we eat. Good nutrition is essential for both keeping a healthy weight and being in good health. It seems that eating habits have just as big of an impact as what and how much we eat.

Meal Plan

Select unprocessed, whole foods:
Whole grains: whole wheat, quinoa, brown rice, and steel-cut oats
veggies (a colorful variety of vegetables, not potatoes)
entire fruits rather than juice
Nuts, seeds, legumes, and other sources of lean protein (fish and poultry)
Plant oils in general, including olive oil
Drink water or other naturally low-calorie beverages.

Don't buy the following things:

sugar-filled drinks (sports drinks, fruit juice, and soda)
Fruit juice (no more than a small amount per day)
Refined grains and sweets include white bread, rice, and pasta.
(Fried or baked) potato
Red meat (beef, hog, and lamb) as well as processed meats like sausage, ham, and bacon

meals that are extensively processed, such as fast food

A well-rounded example of a balanced diet is provided by the Harvard School of Public Health's balanced eating pyramid and healthy eating plate. The Nutrition Source, a companion website to The Obesity Prevention Source, offers a brief guide on choosing healthy drinks in addition to recipes and brief suggestions for healthy eating.

Quantity of Food

A person's daily calorie requirements to either maintain or reduce weight depend on a variety of factors, including age, gender, body type, and level of physical activity. Since two out of every three Americans are overweight or obese, we all need to cut down on our calorie intake.

Online calorie-needs calculators often provide recommendations that are a little bit overly generous. Furthermore, it might be difficult for people to monitor their daily calorie intake in real life.

A better approach is to form eating habits that will keep you from overindulging (see below) and steer clear of foods and beverages that are high in calories and poor in nutrients, such as potatoes, refined carbs, and drinks with added sugar.

How to Quit Overindulging in Food

eat breakfast. While skipping meals may seem like an easy way to cut calories, most of the time it backfires when hunger comes again in the middle of the day, leading to overindulgence.
Consume small amounts of time and slowly. Eating slowly, choosing smaller portions at meals, and giving your brain enough time to tell your stomach when it has had enough food are all possible ways to avoid overindulging. By putting an end to distractions like the internet, smartphones, and television, we can focus on the meal.
Go out to eat. Meals prepared outside the home, such as those from fast food restaurants, often have higher quantities and lower nutritional density than meals prepared at home.

Observe your food. By taking the time to reflect on your initial motivation for eating, you may easily avoid ingesting excess calories. Fed Up? Choose the healthiest menu items and beverages you can. Not really that hungry? Pick something else to do or have a piece of fruit in place of eating the whole meal. To enjoy your food, when you do eat, use all of your senses to completely experience it. More details on mindful eating may be found on the websites of the Center for Mindful Eating and the book Savor Mindful Eating, Mindful Life.

Be Intense

Apart from eating a balanced diet, nothing is more important for keeping a healthy weight and staying in excellent health than frequent exercise. If there was a cure-all for excellent health, it would be exercise.

if you are an adult or a child, and if your goals are to lose weight or maintain good health, will decide how much exercise is recommended. There are several ways to relocate. Select activities you like.

Limiting "sit time" (sedentary time), especially television time, is important for people of all ages. It's also important to remain active.

Guidelines for Physical Activity for Adults:

For optimal health, engage in either 1.25 hours of intense activity (such as jogging or fast cycling) or 2.5 hours of moderate exercise (such as brisk walking or slow riding) every week.

It is advised to engage in moderate-to-intense exercise for one hour each day to help control weight. This workout may be done in quick bursts of ten minutes or more.

Guidelines for Children's Physical Activity:

a minimum of one hour of physical activity every day, divided into shorter bursts of 10 minutes or less.
at least three days a week of bone and muscle building exercises.
These recommendations stress the need to engage children in fun, age-appropriate

activities that encourage increased movement and breathing.

Limit Your Screen Time

Watching television (TV) may be dangerous for your weight even if it can be pleasant and enlightening. Because high-calorie, low-nutrient foods and drinks are often marketed via commercials, product placements, and other types of promotion, this completely sedentary activity also tends to promote unhealthy eating.

To lessen your child's exposure to television and other screen media (such as video games, recreational computer use, and related activities), use the following advice:

All adults:

Don't spend more than two hours a day utilizing screens or watching television. The less, the better.
Guardians:

Children should not watch screens for more than two hours per day. The less, the better.
Underage viewers should not watch any.
Ensure that children's rooms are free of TVs and the Internet.
When eating, avoid watching TV.
Guardians and instructors:

Set limits on the amount of time spent using screens for pleasure.
medical practitioners

Find out from parents how much time their children spend using screens, then provide them tips on cutting that time down.
Become fervent advocates for more stringent regulations on the promotion of children's foods and beverages on television and in the media.
Getting Enough Rest
It's becoming more obvious how important obtaining a good night's sleep is to health, and it may even help with weight management. Although the quantity needed by each person may vary significantly, there is compelling evidence that many adults and children do not

get enough. Here are some recommendations regarding the duration of your sleep.

grownups:

7-8 hours every evening
Little ones:

Children ages 1-3: 12–14 hours per night

3 to 5-year-olds: 11 to 13 hours every night

10–11 hours per night for children aged 5 to 12.

For teenagers, 8.5 to 9.25 hours per night

As a resource, use the National Sleep Foundation

Give kids an advantage.
There is compelling evidence to suggest that a child's early years—including the time spent pregnant—may have a big impact on their weight in the future. Establishing the foundation for excellent health is usually always a smart idea.

With the support of their healthcare providers, women who are of reproductive age, expectant mothers, and new mothers may make decisions that might improve both their own and their children's health.

Advice:

To maintain a healthy weight before becoming pregnant.
Don't smoke when expecting.
Aim for a healthy weight increase throughout pregnancy.
Breastfeed for at least 12 months, preferably for 4 to 6 months without using any other liquids.
As newborns grow into adulthood, make sure they get enough sleep.
Encourage children to gain weight in a healthy way (address during doctor's visits).
Unwind
There are many daily stresses in today's environment. This is a normal part of life, but as stress levels rise, it may lead to poor eating habits and other harmful behaviors that can worsen health and result in weight gain.

Frequent exercise is one of the greatest ways to avoid weight gain and one of the best ways to handle stress. Other mind-body methods, such as breathing exercises, could also be beneficial.

Calculate Your BMI

A person's weight in kilograms divided by their height in meters squared yields their body mass index, or BMI. BMI is a cheap and simple way to test for obesity, overweight, underweight, and healthy weight.

Although body fat is not directly measured by BMI, there is a considerable correlation between BMI and other more direct measurements of body fat. Furthermore, these more precise measurements of body fatness do not seem to have a stronger correlation with other metabolic and disease outcomes than BMI.

Excess body fat may contribute to several health problems and illnesses associated with weight. Underweight poses additional health risks. Waist circumference and body mass index

(BMI) are screening measures used to determine a person's weight status in relation to possible illness risk. Waist circumference and BMI, however, are not diagnostic methods for disease risks. To determine illness status and measure disease risk, a qualified healthcare professional should carry out further health exams.

How to Calculate and Evaluate Your Weight
BMI, or adult body mass index
A person's weight in kilograms divided by their height in meters squared is their BMI. Too little body fatness may be indicated by a low BMI, while too much body fatness can be indicated by a high BMI. Use the BMI Calculator to determine your BMI. Alternatively, use this BMI Index Chart to establish your height and weight and get your BMI.

Your BMI is considered underweight if it is less than 18.5.
Your BMI is within the Healthy Weight range if it is between 18.5 and 24.9.
Your BMI is considered overweight if it is between 25.0 and 29.9.

Your BMI is considered obese if it is 30.0 or greater.
Overweight or obese refers to a weight that exceeds what is deemed healthy for a certain height. Underweight refers to a weight that is less than what is deemed healthy for a certain height.1.

BMI may be used as a screening tool for individuals, but it cannot be used to diagnose a person's health or amount of body fat. To determine a person's health state and dangers, a qualified healthcare professional should conduct the necessary health evaluations.

How to Calculate BMI Using Weight and Height
Measuring weight and height is necessary to determine BMI. Measuring weight in kilos and height in meters gives the most precise results. Nonetheless, the BMI calculation has been modified to account for weight in pounds and height in inches. These measures may be made at home using a tape measure and scale or at the office of a healthcare professional.

Waist Measurement

How to Determine Your Waist Size #2

Position a tape measure slightly above your hipbones around your midsection while standing.
Verify that the tape is horizontal at the waist.
Tighten the tape around your waist without pressuring the skin.
As soon as you release your breath, measure your waist.
Measuring your waist circumference is another technique to determine your possible illness risk. Because it increases your chance of acquiring obesity-related diseases including Type 2 Diabetes, high blood pressure, and coronary artery disease, excess belly fat may be dangerous. If you are one of the following, your waist size may be warning you that you have an increased chance of developing obesity-related conditions:

A guy with a waist size of more than forty inches
A woman who is not pregnant and has a waist circumference of more than 35 inches

Although waist circumference may be used as a screening tool, it cannot be utilized to diagnose a person's body fat or overall health. To determine a person's health state and dangers, a qualified healthcare professional should conduct the necessary health evaluations.

How do you calculate BMI?
The formula for calculating BMI is the same for adults and children. The following formulae form the basis of the calculation:

The formula for calculating BMI is the same for adults and children. The following formulae form the basis of the calculation:

Metric units: kilograms and millimeters
The formula is height (m) / weight (kg).2.

BMI is calculated using the metric system, which is weight in kilograms divided by height in meters squared. Since centimeters are often used to measure height, dividing the height in centimeters by 100 will give you the height in meters.

For instance, 68 kg of weight and 165 cm (1.65 m) of height
68 ÷ (1.65)2 = 24.98 is the calculation.

Inches and pounds
Weight (lb) / [height (in)]2×703 is the formula.

By dividing weight in pounds (lbs) by height in inches (in) squared, and multiplying the result by 703, you may get your BMI.

Example: 5'5 (65") tall, 150 pounds of weight
[150 ÷ (65)2] x 703 = 24.96 is the calculation.

How is an adult's BMI interpreted?
Standard weight status categories are used to interpret BMI for people 20 years of age and older. Men and women of all ages and physical kinds fall into the same groups.
The following table displays the standard weight status categories corresponding to adult BMI ranges.

Body mass index (kg/m²)	Weight condition
Below 18.5	Underweight
18.5 to 24.9	Healthy weight
25.0 to 29.9	Overweight
30.0 and above	Obesity

For an individual who is 5′ 9″ tall, for instance, these are the weight ranges, matching BMI ranges, and weight status categories.

Height	Weight range (lbs)	BMI	Weight condition
5' 9"	124 or less	Below 18	Underweight
	125 to 168	18.5 to 24.9	Healthy weight
	168 to 202	25.0 to 29.9	Overweight

	203 and above	30 or higher	Obesity

Even though BMI for children and teenagers is computed using the same method as BMI for adults, it is interpreted differently. Because body fat levels vary across genders and alter with age, BMIs for children and teenagers must take these factors into account. These variations are taken into consideration in the CDC BMI-for-age growth charts, which graphically represent BMI as a percentile ranking. These percentiles were calculated using representative data from surveys conducted between 1963–1965 and 1988–1941, which covered the 2- to 19-year-old population in the US.

A BMI of 2 to 19 years old that is at or above the 95th percentile of children of the same age and sex in this reference group from 1963 to 1994 is considered obese. For instance, a 10-year-old boy weighing 102 pounds and with an average height of 56 inches would have a BMI of 22.9 kg/m2. The youngster would be classified as obese as his BMI would be in the 95th percentile, which is higher than the BMIs of 95% of boys in this reference sample who are similarly aged.

Generally speaking, women have higher body fat percentages than males do at the same BMI. Depending on the racial/ethnic group, the percentage of body fat may vary at the same BMI 13–15.
Generally speaking, older folks have higher body fat percentages than younger ones with the same BMI.
Athletes have lower body fat percentages than non-athletes at the same BMI.
Those with greater BMI and body fatness levels also seem to have better accuracy levels for BMI as an indication of body fatness16. Although a person with a very high BMI (35 kg/m2) is most certainly obese, a somewhat high BMI may also indicate a high proportion of lean body mass (bone and muscle). To determine a person's health state and dangers, a qualified healthcare professional should conduct the necessary health evaluations.

Is someone still deemed overweight if they are an athlete or another person with a high body mass index yet their BMI is above 25?
Anybody with a BMI between 25 and 29.9 would be considered overweight, and anybody with a BMI above 30 would be considered obese, according to the BMI weight status classifications.

Nonetheless, rather than having more body fat, athletes may have a high BMI due to enhanced muscularity. Although this may not apply to athletes, a person with a high BMI is generally thought to be overweight or obese and to have body fat. To determine a person's health state and dangers, a qualified healthcare professional should conduct the necessary health evaluations.

Recipes for Breakfast

You must have the energy to get out of bed in the morning in order to have a great day. That should include a nutritious, well-balanced breakfast in addition to your usual cup of coffee.

The phrase "part of a balanced breakfast" has undoubtedly been heard in many cereal advertisements. Breakfast is one of the most essential meals of the day, as we have often been reminded. The adverts did not, however, explain what precisely constitutes a healthy, balanced breakfast (apart from those sugary cereals, evidently).

Studies have shown that meals rich in protein, such as eggs and chicken sausage, are preferable to those heavy in carbs, such as cereals. Getting enough protein in your diet at the beginning of the day can help you feel full and satisfied all day. Breakfasts high in protein may also assist you in making better decisions throughout the rest of the day. A 2023 research indicated that eating a high-protein breakfast reduced the likelihood of grabbing high-fat or high-sugar snacks later in the day. This helps manage blood sugar and insulin levels. The study was published in the American Journal of Clinical Nutrition. In addition to reducing your chance of acquiring diabetes, this may also lessen your cravings.

You can't be intended to consume exclusively protein in the morning, can you?

Correct. Protein and fiber are equally vital for a healthy start to the day. Additionally, it may help you feel full after a meal and prevent you from reaching for empty calories during snack time. Additionally, the vitamin has been connected to a decreased incidence of fatal illnesses.

For maximum muscle growth and maintenance advantages, Men's Health generally suggests eating 30 grams of protein and 10 grams of fiber at each meal. These meals are going to help you get there. Moreover, they taste great. Thus, you may feed your weight reduction with more than just eggs and chicken sausage.

And it's particularly fortunate because boredom is one thing that should never be a part of breakfast. To start the day off correctly, try these alternatives.

1. Migas

Are you a fan of breakfast? Are you a Nacho fan? Then have these nachos for breakfast in the morning. They are crisp. They are floppy. They are corny. They're also excellent for finishing up the tortilla chip shake that's left in the bag's bottom.

What is required:
Tbsp canola oil
1/4 chopped medium white onion (about half a cup)
one cup of tortilla chips, gently crushed
Three big eggs

Two tablespoons of shredded cheddar or pepper jack cheese
Half an avocado, diced
one-third cup of black beans
two or three stalks of cilantro leaves
To taste, hot sauce

Methods:
1. Heat the canola oil in a large nonstick pan over medium heat. Add the onion and simmer for 2 to 3 minutes, stirring periodically, until transparent. Add the chips and cook for approximately two minutes, or until aromatic. After that, break in the eggs, reduce the heat to medium-low, and cook for one to two minutes, stirring frequently, until the eggs set.
Place the migas on a big platter and garnish with the spicy sauce, cheese, beans, avocado, and cilantro.

dietary information
30 g protein, 41 g carbs, 11 g fiber, and 50 g fat make up the 732 calories.

2. Avocado Salsa and Black Bean Huevos Rancheros

When huevos appear on a restaurant menu, people usually become very excited about them. Justifiably so, since they're excellent. Unless, of course, you're sitting at your dining room table and it's not that hard to wig out about them either. Allow this to cook for ten minutes. Consume. Enrage. Think of starting your own eatery.

Requirements: 1/2 cup washed and drained canned black beans
1/2 diced avocado and 1/4 chopped tiny red onion
1/4 lime's worth of juice
Chop 1 tablespoon of cilantro.
Tbsp canola oil
Two petite (6-inch) flour tortillas
two eggs

Methods: 1. Combine the black beans, avocado, onion, lime juice, and cilantro in a medium-sized bowl. Use salt and pepper to season to taste.
2. Heat the canola oil in a small, nonstick pan over medium heat. Add the tortillas piled on top

of each other when the oil begins to shimmer. Cook for 15 to 30 seconds or until the top tortilla puffs up. Flip the stack and then the top tortilla using tongs. Until the tortillas are cooked on both sides, repeat step 4 four more times. Place the tortillas onto a dish for dishing. 3. Reduce the heat to medium-low in the pan. Gently crack in the eggs, place a lid on the pan, and simmer for 2 to 4 minutes, or until the whites are set. After slipping the eggs onto the tortillas, cover them with salsa. Use a knife and fork to eat.

Dietary Information
671 calories, 39 g fat, 60 g carbs, 26 g protein, and 13 g fiber

3. Peanut-butter oatmeal and black-cherry shake

A 5-year study of 86,000 physicians found that men who consumed at least one dish of whole-grain cereal (like oatmeal) a day had the lowest chance of dying from any cause, including heart disease. Because salicylates, the active component of aspirin, are found naturally in cherries and strawberries, they are excellent natural remedies for morning headaches brought on by stress.

What is required:
1 cup of juiced cherries
One cup of strawberries, frozen
One cup of frozen cherries without sugar
Two tsp of protein powder
1/3 cup of oats
1 tablespoon peanut butter
half a cup of milk

Method: Using a blender, blend the protein powder, frozen fruit, and cherry juice until smooth. Follow the instructions on the box to microwave the oatmeal. Add the milk and peanut butter and stir. Shakes once.

dietary information
    600 calories, 10 g fiber, 100 g carbs, 27 g protein, and 11 g fat

4. rotein Oats for Overnight

This is the ideal one-minute meal for a man who works out in the morning.

What You'll Need: ½ cup old-fashioned rolled oats
½ cup of milk
Choco protein powder, 2 tablespoons
One banana, cut.
Half a cup of blueberries

How to Make It: Combine the oats, milk, and protein powder in a dish or jar. Refrigerate overnight with a cover on. Simply remove the cover and microwave the oats for one minute in the morning. Incorporate the fruit and savor.

dietary information
432 calories, 22g fat, 72g carbohydrates, 9g fiber, and 9g protein.

5. Sappy Morning Roll-Up
This quick and simple recipe relies on melted edam cheese to bring everything together.

What is required:
1 teaspoon canola oil

four cherry tomatoes cut up
One tablespoon finely sliced red onion
1/2 chopped jalapeño
one little clove of chopped garlic
two eggs
Single whole-wheat tortilla
One handful of Edam cheese crumbles

How to Make It: Heat the oil in a small pan over medium heat. Add the garlic, onion, jalapeño, tomatoes, and a little amount of salt. For approximately two minutes, stir to coat and sizzle until melted. After that, add the eggs, stir well to break up the yolk, and cook for a further two minutes or until scrambled. Stir to partially melt the cheese before adding it to the tortilla. Roll up to consume.

dietary information
435 calories, 28g fat, 25g carbohydrates, 9g fiber, and 17g protein.

6. Toasted Salmon
If you love lox on a bagel, you should try this healthier version of the traditional morning dish.

dish at an outside restaurant with starters

Two pieces of whole-wheat bread are required.
Two tsp of cream cheese
Two-ounce smoked salmon
One tablespoon of capers
Dill, for flavor
Red onion, flavor-wise
Lemon extract
One pear

How to Produce It

Top two ounces of smoked salmon, one tablespoon of capers, a little finely sliced red onion, fresh lemon juice, and some fresh dill over two slices of whole-wheat bread spread with two tablespoons of cream cheese. Enjoy with a medium-sized, juicy pear.

dietary information
55 g carbohydrates, 10 g fiber, 19 g fat, 45 g protein, and 551 calories

7. Yogurt Bowl

If you want a sweet breakfast, eating a lot of fruit is a terrific way to get all the taste. Berries are also a fantastic source of sweetness and fiber.

1 1/2 cups of plain, 2% Greek yogurt are required.
One-fourth cup blueberries
One-fourth cup raspberries
one-fourth cup strawberries
One-fourth cup blackberries
Bite-sized pistachios
flakes of coconut without sugar

How to Create It: Best Combine 1 1/2 cups of plain 2% Greek yogurt with 1/4 cup of each of the following: unsweetened coconut flakes, unsalted dry-roasted shelled pistachios, sliced strawberries, blackberries, blueberries, and raspberries.

dietary information

621 calories, 37g fat, 43g carbohydrates, 11g fiber, and 36g protein

8. Hash Turkey

This is a really hearty breakfast to have after Thanksgiving.

Requirements: 1 tablespoon of olive oil
4 ounces of turkey breast, cut finely
1/4 minced onion, 1 small chopped zucchini, and 1 big diced potato
One cup of Brussels sprouts, shredded
fiery sauce

How to Make It: Saute 1 cup shredded Brussels sprouts, 1/4 minced onion, 1 small chopped zucchini, and 4 ounces of finely chopped leftover turkey breast in 1 tablespoon olive oil. Add plenty of spicy sauce on top.

dietary information
640 calories, 81 g carbohydrates, 10 g fiber, 16 g fat, and 47 g protein.

9. Breakfast Fish from Bermuda? Hey, give it a try before you judge it.

Ingredients: 4 ounces of roasted cod
2 tablespoons warm salsa
One big russet potato, coarsely diced, served with broiled fries
1/4 avocado, sliced
one egg, hardboiled

How to Make It: Top 4 ounces of roasted fish served with 1 big broiled russet potato, coarsely diced, and 2 tablespoons of warmed salsa on the side. Present a quarter of an avocado sliced and a hard-boiled egg beside. Ignore the conventional banana.

dietary information
10 g fiber, 16 g fat, 75 g carbohydrates, 36 g protein, and 579 calories

10. Egg Scramble With Sweet Potatoes
If you can scramble some eggs, you can scramble some eggs while you roast some sweet potatoes.

What You'll Need:
8 oz diced sweet potato
1/2 cup chopped onion
2 tsp chopped fresh rosemary
Cooking spray
4 large eggs
4 large egg whites
2 Tbsp chopped fresh chives

How to Make It:
1. Preheat your oven to 425°F. On a baking sheet, toss the sweet potato, onion, rosemary, 1/4 each tsp salt and pepper. Lightly coat the vegetables with cooking spray then roast until tender, about 20 minutes.
2. Meanwhile, in a small bowl, whisk the eggs and egg whites, and season with a pinch each of salt and pepper. Coat a large skillet with cooking spray and then heat over medium. Add the eggs and cook, stirring frequently, until scrambled, 3 to 4 minutes. Sprinkle the eggs, potatoes, and onions, with chives. Feeds 1

Nutritional facts
571 calories, 44 g protein, 52 g carbs, 9 g fiber, 20 g fat

11. PB Protein Overnight Oatmeal

Never underestimate the power of adding a scoop of protein powder to something other than a shake—especially oatmeal.

What You'll Need:
1/2 cup steel-cut oats
2 Tbsp peanut butter
1 scoop (35g) chocolate protein powder
1/2 sliced banana
1 Tbsp raisins
1 Tbsp chopped walnuts

How to Make It:
1. In a small saucepan over medium heat, add the oats, a pinch of salt, and 1 1/3 cups water. Bring to a simmer, and then remove the pan from the heat. Stir in the peanut butter. Cover, refrigerate, and let the oats soak overnight.
2. In the morning, stir in the protein powder. Heat the oatmeal over medium-low for 5 minutes, stirring a couple times, until heated

through. Transfer to bowls, then top with banana, raisins, and walnuts. Feeds 3

Nutritional facts
740 calories, 42 g protein, 84 g carbs, 13 g fiber, 28 g fat

12. Tropical-Powered Oatmeal Bowl

If you're sick of bananas and raisins, shake things up a bit, with this protein-powder-reinforced breakfast.

What You'll Need:
½ cup old-fashioned oats
1 scoop vanilla protein powder
2 Tbsp heavy cream
1 tsp vanilla extract
½ mango, sliced
½ star fruit, sliced
½ cup pineapple, cubed
2 Tbsp pomegranate seeds
2 Tbsp unsweetened coconut flakes
Torn mint leaves

How to Make It:

In a bowl, mix the oats with 1 cup water and pinch of salt. Microwave for 2 ½ minutes. Stir in the protein powder, cream, and extract. Top with the remaining ingredients.

Nutritional facts
646 calories, 34 g protein, 72 g carbs, 10 g fiber, 24 g fat

13. Almond Banana Shake
Yeah, a shake can be a solid breakfast too. Just make sure you're hitting your goal of at least 30 grams of protein and 10 grams of fiber and you're good to go.

What You'll Need:
1 cup coconut water
1 cup plain Greek yogurt
6 tbsp almond butter
2 scoops whey protein powder
2 Tbsp hulled hemp seeds
1 Tbsp chia seeds
2 frozen banana
2 cup ice

How to Make It:

In a blender, pulverize all the ingredients till smooth, adding additional coconut water to adjust consistency, if needed.

Nutritional facts
    714 calories, 42 g protein, 64 g carbs, 10 g fiber, 17 g fat

    14. Chocolate Cherry Power Shake
And, if you're more of a chocolate guy, here's this stunner.

What You'll Need:
1/2 cup frozen cherries
8 oz water
1/2 cup chopped raw beets
1/2 cup frozen strawberries
1/2 cup frozen blueberries
1/2 banana
1 scoop chocolate whey protein
2 Tbsp chia seeds

How to Make It:
In a blender, pulverize all the ingredients till smooth, adding additional water to adjust consistency, if needed.

Nutritional facts
429 calories, 30 g protein, 4 g fat, 52 g carbs, 10 g fiber, 11 g fiber

15. Blueberry Vanilla Breakfast Shake
Maybe you're a vanilla fan instead. We got you.

What You'll Need:
1 cup blueberries
1/2 banana
1 1/2 scoops vanilla protein powder
2 Tbsp walnuts
2 Tbsp oats
1 Tbsp chia seeds

How to Make It:
In a blender, pulverize all the ingredients till smooth, adding water to adjust consistency, if needed.

Nutritional facts
536 calories, 42 g protein, 59 g carbs, 12 g fiber, 18 g fat

16. Spicy Avocado Sourdough Toast and Eggs

There's a reason there's avocado toast is having a moment. Try it out.

What You'll Need:
2 slices of Ezekiel whole grain bread
1 egg
1/2 cup egg whites
Half an avocado
Hot sauce of your choice
Red pepper flakes, to taste

How To Make It:
Toast the bread. Make the eggs however you like them best— but we like them scrambled. Smear half an avocado on the toast, add desired amount of red pepper flakes on top. Top with the eggs when done, add however much hot sauce you want depending on how spicy you like it!

Nutritional facts
368 calories, 25 g protein, 37 g carbs, 10 g fiber, 11 g fat

17. Greek Toast and Eggs

You've heard of avocado toast, but have you heard of hummus toast? Now you have.

What You'll Need:
2 slices of Ezekiel whole grain bread
1 egg
1/2 cup egg whites
2 oz of feta crumbles
2 Tbsp hummus, plain or flavor of your choice

How To Make It:
Toast the bread. Make the eggs however you like—but we like them scrambled. Season them as you like. We like adding a little bit of steak seasoning to them. Smear the hummus on the toast. Top with the eggs and feta crumbles.

Nutritional facts
400 calories, 38 g protein, 42 g carbs, 10 g fiber, 17 g fat

18. Turkey Bacon and Mozzarella Breakfast Burrito

You're welcome.

What You'll Need:
1 egg
1/2 cup egg whites
1 carb balance tortilla
4 slices turkey bacon
1/4 cup mozzarella
1 cup spinach
Hot sauce, to taste

How To Make It:
Preheat the oven to 400°F. Make the eggs and egg whites however you like—but we like them scrambled. Season them as you like. While those are cooking, throw the turkey bacon in the oven for 10 minutes, each side. Assemble put your eggs, bacon, and spinach onto your tortilla. Top with the mozzarella and hot sauce for a bit of spice. Roll into a burrito.

Nutritional facts
442 calories, 47 g protein, 25 g carbs, 16 g fiber, 22 g fat

19. Customizable Egg Cups

You've seen the egg cups at Starbucks. These will pack the protein, and veggies and a side of fruit will contribute your much needed fiber. The best part is you can customize them to your liking: choose different high-fiber vegetables and fruits to switch it up, and season as you please.

What You'll Need:

4 eggs

1/2 cup of egg whites

2 links of low fat chicken sausage

1/2 cup of broccoli or carrots

1 cup of raspberries or blackberries

How to Make It:

Mix eggs, egg whites, veggies, and cut up chicken sausage into a bowl and mix. Distribute evenly into a muffin tin, making sure you get equal amounts of sausage into each tin. Bake at 350 degrees for 20 mins.

Nutritional facts

For 3 muffins and a side of raspberries: 335 calories, 25.5 g protein, 16 g fat, 15 g carbs, 10 g fiber

20.   Protein-Packed Breakfast PB&J

For a "nostalgic" and "nutrient-dense" breakfast, Melanie Murphy Richter, M.S., R.D.N., and instructor of nutrition physiology at University of California Irvine suggests this spin on an old classic. This meal "supports muscle synthesis and sustained energy throughout the day," she says.

What You'll Need:

½ cup of fresh mixed berries

1 Tbsp of honey

1 Tbsp of chia seeds

3 Tbsp of peanut butter

two slices of sprouted Ezekiel bread

1 Tbsp of hemp hearts

How to Make It:

Mash fresh mixed berries with honey and chia seeds until it's a nice jelly consistency. Then spread around three tablespoons of peanut butter on two slices of sprouted Ezekiel bread, and top it with your jelly mixture plus one tablespoon of hemp hearts.

Nutritional facts
Per serving (2 pieces of toast): 500 calories, 35g fat, 50g carbs, 15g fiber, 25g protein

Important Salads

How to Pick the Healthiest Salad Ingredients to Help You Lose Weight

Use these suggestions to choose the salad elements that can help you lose weight:

1. Select Variously Colored Vegetables

Don't limit yourself to simply green veggies; a variety of vitamins and minerals are found in various colored vegetables, and our bodies need them all. Along with your greens, add some red (tomatoes, bell peppers, etc.), white (mushrooms, shallots, etc.), orange (carrots, squashes, etc.), purple (eggplant, cabbage, etc.), and other similar veggies.

2. Include Meat

Add proteins like fish (tuna, shrimp, etc.), meat (grilled chicken, lean steak, etc.), or grains (brown rice, barley, etc.) to your diet to prolong feeling full.

3. Include Good Fats

In addition to vitamins, minerals, and protein, our bodies also need a reasonable amount of lipids. Choose fats that are healthier than ones that won't aid in weight reduction. Nuts (almonds, walnuts, pine nuts, etc.), seeds (chia seeds, pumpkin seeds, etc.), and olive oil are a few healthy choices.

4. Select a Nutritious Base

Avoid using potatoes or pasta as the foundation of your salad as they may be heavy in fat and calories. Make sure there are more greens in your foundation. Add more sharper greens, such as lettuce, cabbage, and other vegetables, and less spring greens, such as mustard greens, spinach, chard, etc.

5. Use a nutritious salad dressing

Your favorite gourmet shop has a plethora of selections, but keep in mind that most of these dressings are rich in calories. Making your own dressing using olive oil, citrus fruits, spices, salt, and pepper is thus your best option.

6. Select the Proper Herbs
Go for locally accessible, fresh, in-season herbs
rather than dried ones. A dried herb cannot
provide the flavor and scent that fresh herbs
may provide to a salad. You have a wide variety
of herbs to pick from, including thyme, basil,
dill, and rosemary.

Top Recipes for Weight Loss Salads
Here are a broad range of salad recipes that are
sure to please everyone and may aid in weight
loss:

1.   A salad with spinach and cabbage
This quick and simple green salad dish doesn't
need to be cooked; it can be put together
quickly.

Components

Distilled spinach greens, ½ cup
Half a cup of shredded cabbage
½ cup of red cabbage shredded
Two tablespoons of chopped walnuts and ½
cup of thickly shredded carrots

two tsp lemon juice
1 tablespoon coarsely minced garlic and ¼ teaspoon mustard powder
1/2 tsp black pepper
Add salt to taste. Cook for 10 to 15 minutes total.

Ninety-nine calories

Servings: four to six

How to Produce

Give every vegetable a thorough wash.
Combine all the salad ingredients in a large bowl. Discard it completely.
Serve right away.

2. Salad of sprouts
The process of tempering intensifies the crunchiness of the veggies and pulses while also enhancing their flavor. You can quickly prepare this sprout salad dish to help you lose weight.

Components

One cup of mixed sprouts (chana, rajma, moong daal, etc.)

¼ cup grated radish; ½ cup chopped tomatoes; 2 tsp chopped coriander; ¼ cup chopped, coarsely chopped methi leaves; 1 chopped green chili

A tsp oil and a pinch of hing

Add salt to taste.

Cooking time total: 12 to 15 minutes

50 calories are included.

Servings: four to six

How to Produce

Combine all the ingredients listed above in a large bowl, except the oil, hing, and green chili. Throw them politely.

Heat some oil in a skillet, then add the green chili and hing, and sauté for a little while.

Over the sprout salad, pour the tempering, toss to combine, and serve.

3. Bean Sprout with Capsicum Salad
The abundant vitamin C content of both the bean sprouts and the capsicum makes this salad dish a vitamin C powerhouse.

Components

1 ½ cups bean sprouts and ¼ cup thinly sliced capsicum
1 tsp coarsely chopped garlic
1 teaspoon soy sauce
two tsp vinegar
A tsp of chili powder
1/4 tsp sugar
1 ½ tablespoons of coarsely crushed roasted peanuts
½ teaspoon oil
One tablespoon of chopped spring onions

Cooking time total: 12–15 minutes

60 calories

Servable: 3–4

How to Produce

Combine the soy sauce, vinegar, sugar, peanuts, and chili powder in a bowl. Put away.
Garlic is added to hot oil and sautéed for a brief period of time. Allow to cool.
Combine the bean sprouts, capsicum, and both dressings, mixing well.
Add some chopped spring onions as a garnish and serve.

4. A salad of vegetables and sprouts
This salad recipe's nutritious value is enhanced by the addition of sprouts.

Components

½ cup of mixed boiling sprouts, such as moong daal, rajma, and kala chana.

One cup of coarsely chopped lettuce
one cup of cubed capsicum
½ tbsp lemon juice and 1 tablespoon minced
spring onions
½ cup low-fat curd
Add pepper and salt to taste.

Fry Time in Total: 15 minutes

45 calories

Servable: 3–4

How to Produce

Combine curd, lemon juice, salt, and pepper in
a bowl. Put aside.
Combine all the salad ingredients in a large
bowl and mix well.
Let it cool for one hour. Present cold.

5. Pickled Kale
This salad is high in vitamin C, vitamin A, and
fiber. Crunchy cucumbers are given a tart edge
by the luscious red tomatoes.

Components
One cup of sliced cucumber, two cups of iceberg lettuce, coarsely shredded, and two cups of deseeded, chopped, and cubed tomatoes
One tablespoon of basil leaves
1 tsp smashed garlic and 2 tsp lemon juice
1 teaspoon olive oil

Cooking Time in Total: 10 Min
60 calories
4 servings

How to Produce
Mix well after combining all of the components listed above.
Serve right away.

6. Salad with corn, broccoli, and jalapeños
The salad's high fiber content fills you up and gives you the energy you really need.

Components
One-third cup of cooked corn kernels

3 cups florets of broccoli
½ cup chopped onions, 1 tablespoon chopped jalapeño, and 1 teaspoon olive oil
Add salt to taste.

Cooking Time in Total: 10 Min
90 calories
4 servings

How to Produce
Put the steamed broccoli aside.
In a skillet with heated oil, sauté onions over medium heat for a few minutes.
Add the broccoli, corn, jalapeño, and salt; sauté for two to three minutes over high heat.
Warm up the food.

7. Salad of Watermelon

Watermelon is an ingredient in this fruit salad dish that helps you feel satiated for longer.

Components:
One large dish of cubed watermelon
one cup of pitted black olives

200 grams of feta cheese, finely chopped with a few mint leaves and bite-sized chunks
1 small onion, finely diced; 4 tablespoons olive oil
to taste, black pepper

Cooking Time in Total: 10 Min
80 calories
Servable: 3–4

How to Produce
Combine the watermelon, feta cheese, onions, mint leaves, and black olives in a large bowl.
After thoroughly mixing with some black pepper and olive oil, serve.

8. Veggie Quinoa Salad
This delicious dish for kala chana salad provides you with extra protein in addition to being satisfying.

Components
Boil two cups of kala chana
1 teaspoon mustard seeds
Minimal curry leaves and ½ tsp black pepper
1 tablespoon lemon juice

One teaspoon oil
Add salt to taste.

Cooking Time in Total: 10 Min
150 calories
4 servings

How to Produce
In a non-stick pan, heat the oil.
Add curry leaves and mustard seeds.
Stir in the lemon juice, salt, pepper, and cooked
chana. Fry for two to three minutes.
Warm up the food.

9. Salad with Chickpeas.

Packed with essential minerals and vitamins,
protein, and dietary fiber, this salad might be a
great choice for lunch if you're attempting to
lose weight.

Components
Boil two cups of chickpeas
One peeled and diced tiny cucumber; one chopped onion; one chopped tomato; and two teaspoons of lemon juice
Mint chutney, 2 to 3 tablespoons
A smidgeon of cumin powder
1/4 tsp powdered black pepper

Cooking time total: 10–12 minutes
145 calories
4 servings

How to Produce
Toss the boiling chickpeas, onions, cucumbers, and tomatoes in a large salad dish.
Add the pepper, cumin, and mint chutney powders along with the lemon juice. Assist.

10. Blend a salad of vegetables.
With the least amount of work, this weight loss dish for mixed vegetable salad is created.

Components

One cup chopped capsicum, one cup diced cucumber, and one-and-a-half cups cubed carrots
A few spinach leaves, coarsely ripped ½ cup shredded cabbage leaves and two teaspoons of lemon juice
To taste, add salt and black pepper.

Cooking time total: 10–15 minutes
55 calories
Servable: 3–4

How to Produce
Place all the chopped vegetables in a bowl and stir well.
Add the pepper, salt, and lemon juice. After fully combining, serve.

11. Carrot and Pomegranate Salad

For those who like a hint of sweetness, this dish for weight reduction fruit and vegetable salad is perfect.

Components
cup of pomegranates
Cup of julienned carrots
a few finely cut mint leaves
Two tsp of lemon juice
One teaspoon of brown sugar, one teaspoon of rock salt, and one teaspoon of black pepper

Cooking time total: 15-20 minutes
65 calories
3 servings

How to Produce
Grab a big bowl. Incorporate the lemon juice, sugar, rock salt, black pepper, and mint leaves. Blend well.
Add carrots and pomegranates. After a good stir, serve.

Q&As
The following are some common queries:

1. Will I Gain Weight If I Eat Too Much Salad?
Even though most salads include fresh fruit and green vegetables, eating too much salad is not advised since it might hinder your efforts to lose weight, particularly if the salad has a lot of dressing or high-calorie add-ons.

2. Can I Lose Weight By Eating Salad Alone?
The ingredients in your salad may have an impact on how much weight you lose. So, in addition to leading a healthy lifestyle, pay attention to what goes into your salad. Steer clear of high-calorie condiments like cheese, creams, sauces, and other items that might cause weight gain rather than loss.

Simplify your diet with these delicious and easy salad dishes to shed pounds in a healthy manner!

The Veggies

Simple Healthy Vegetable Recipes to Help You Lose Weight

Have you been trying to find a way to support yourself while losing weight? These are a few nutritious vegetable salad recipes that might help you lose weight.

1. Sandwich with Hummus and Veggies

This is a great on-the-go vegetarian weight reduction snack that is heart-healthy. You can also make it more interesting by combining various vegetable varieties with hummus tastes. Here's how to prepare sandwiches with vegetables and hummus:

Two slices of whole-grain bread are the ingredients;

3 tsp hummus and ¼ mashed avocado

Half a cup of mixed green salad

a half-cup of cucumber slices

half a cup of carrot shreds
Guidelines:
Begin by spreading hummus on one piece of bread and mashed avocado on the other.
Next, add bell pepper, cucumber, carrots, and greens to the sandwich.
After cutting the sandwich in half, serve it.

2. Caramelized Noodles

Due to its very healthful monounsaturated fats, peanut butter is essential to any diet plan aimed at weight reduction. Ginger may boost your metabolism and make you feel fuller for longer, which is an extra benefit. To create peanut butter noodles, follow these steps:

Ingredients: a quarter of a cup of peanut butter
One-third cup of soy sauce
One-third cup agave sweetener
Twice as much water
one tablespoon finely chopped ginger
one minced garlic clove
A quarter-tsp apple cider vinegar
Sesame oil, one teaspoonful
a half-tongue of Sriracha
Soba noodles, 4 ounces

¾ cup of cucumbers, cut into ribbons
One scallion, diced
1/4 cup of peanuts (optional) as a garnish
One diced scallion, optional for garnish
Guidelines:
To make the sauce, start by mixing the first nine components. Now carefully mix them until they are smooth and properly combined.
Next, prepare the soba noodles according to the package's instructions, and as soon as you take them from the stove, immediately cover them with cold water.
Allow to cool for 20 to 30 seconds. When the noodles are cold, rinse them and toss them with the sauce, cucumber, and scallions.
If desired, garnish with peanuts.

3. Curry Soup with Roasted Cauliflower and Potatoes

Roasting the cauliflower in this dish keeps the florets from becoming too soft while adding depth of flavor. The soup has a thick, creamy texture from the coconut milk and a little amount of tomato sauce. Serve it with some yogurt or sour cream. This is how to prepare soup with roasted cauliflower and potatoes:

Ingredients
- Two tablespoons of ground coriander are the.
- One and a half tablespoons of ground cinnamon and two teaspoons of cumin
- one-half teaspoon of turmeric powder
- A quarter-tsp salt
- A quarter-tsp of ground pepper
- One-half teaspoon of cayenne
- One small head of cauliflower, chopped into roughly six cups of tiny florets
- Two teaspoons of extra virgin olive oil, divided
- one big onion, chopped
- One cup of chopped carrots and three big minced garlic cloves
- 1 ½ teaspoon freshly grated ginger
- One freshly chopped serrano or jalapeño red chili pepper, plus more for garnish
- One 14-ounce can of tomato sauce without additional salt
- Low-sodium vegetable broth in four cups

- Three cups of russet potatoes, chopped and skinned (1/2 inch)
- Two tablespoons of lime juice and two teaspoons of lime zest
- One fourteen-ounce can of coconut milk
- chopped cilantro, fresh, for garnish
-

Directions:
- Preheat the oven to about 450 degrees Fahrenheit.
- Next, in a separate bowl, mix together the cumin, cinnamon, coriander, turmeric, pepper, salt, and cayenne.
- Add the cauliflower to a large bowl along with 1 tablespoon of oil. Toss again after adding 1 tablespoon of the spice mixture to the bowl. Arrange it on a rimmed baking sheet in a single layer.
- Once the cauliflower's edges are browned, roast it for 15 to 20 minutes, then remove and put aside.
- Next, heat the last tablespoon of oil in a big saucepan over medium-high heat.
- To cook, add the onion and carrots. For approximately 3 to 4 minutes, or until

they become brown, make careful to stir often. Add the ginger, garlic, chili, and remaining spice combination. Cook, stirring, for a little more than a minute.

- Scrape up any browned parts and stir in the tomato sauce. Simmer for one minute.
- Add the lime zest and juice, sweet potatoes, and soup. Place a lid on the mixture and heat it to a boiling point.
- Lower the temperature to maintain a low simmer and cook with a partly covered dish. When the veggies are soft, continue stirring them every 35 to 40 minutes.
- Incorporate the roasted cauliflower and coconut milk into the mixture. Bring back to a simmer to finish heating.
- Garnish with chilies and cilantro, if preferred.

4. Cheesy Spaghetti Squash Stuffed with Spinach and Artichokes

This recipe offers you a deliciously creamy dish with a significant reduction in calories.

Roasting the squash will bring forth its greatest taste. This is how you succeed:

Ingredients:
3 tablespoons split water, one 2 ½ to 3 pounds of spaghetti squash sliced in half lengthwise with all of its seeds removed
One box (5 ounces) of baby spinach
Four ounces of reduced-fat cream cheese, cubed and softened; one 10-ounce bag of frozen artichoke hearts, thawed and diced.
½ cup of split grated Parmesan cheese; ¼ teaspoon each of salt and ground pepper
Crushed red pepper and finely chopped fresh basil as garnish

Guidelines:
- In a microwave-safe dish, place the squash cut-side down and add 2 tablespoons of water.
- Now, microwave it for ten to fifteen minutes on high, covered.
- In a large skillet set over medium heat, combine the spinach with the remaining water.

- Simmer for 3 to 5 minutes, stirring periodically, or until wilted.
- Next, scrape any squash from the shells into the basin using a fork. These shells should be put on a baking pan.
- Incorporate the squash mixture with the cream cheese, artichoke hearts, salt, pepper, and ¼ cup of Parmesan cheese. The cheese should become golden brown after three minutes under the broiler.
- If preferred, garnish with chopped basil and crushed pepper.

CHICKEN RECIPE

1. Sandwich Made With Grilled Chicken and Chimichurri Sauce

NUTRITION: 475 mg of sodium, 8 g of fat (3 g saturated), and 310 calories

4 SERVES

You'll need

Four skinless, boneless chicken thighs, six ounces each

To taste, add salt and black pepper.

two cups of assorted infant greens

Four sesame-filled whole-wheat buns, divided and gently toasted

1/2 red onion, cut thinly

1/2 cup of roasted red peppers from a jar

half a cup of chimichurri

METHODS TO BEGIN

- Heat a cast-iron skillet, grill pan, or barbecue.
- After applying salt and pepper to all sides of the chicken, grill or sear it for 3 to 4 minutes on each side, or until it is cooked through and firm.
- Spoon the combined greens onto each bottom bun.
- Place a chicken thigh on top of each sandwich and then heap on the peppers and onion.
- After adding the chimichurri, cover with the remaining bread halves.

Suck This Advice

You can get red peppers that have been roasted in a bottle at any store, but why not roast them yourself to save some money? Cook the bell peppers (red and yellow work best) at 400°F for approximately 25 minutes, or until the skin becomes black and the flesh becomes tender. You may also cook them on a grill or even on a gas burner over moderate heat. After putting the peppers in a dish and covering them with plastic wrap, let them alone for ten minutes.

Peel off the black skin by removing the plastic wrap; this is made simple by the steam produced when the peppers are covered. They are ready to consume after discarding the seeds and stalks.

2. Thai Chicken Spiced with Basil

NUTRITION: 6 g fat (1.5 g saturated), 890 mg salt, and 190 calories

4 SERVES
You'll need
1 tablespoon canola or peanut oil
One medium red onion cut thinly
Thinly slice two jalapeño peppers (or more, if you prefer your cuisine particularly spicy).
four minced garlic cloves
One pound of skinless, boneless chicken breasts, sliced into little pieces
Two tablespoons of fish sauce (If you can't locate fish sauce at all, you can make a similar-tasting version using extra low-sodium

soy sauce and a splash of Worcestershire sauce.)

1 teaspoon sugar

A tablespoon of low-sodium soy sauce

Two cups of fresh basil leaves (holy or Thai basil, which are available mainly at specialized stores)

METHODS TO BEGIN

- In a big skillet or wok, heat the oil.
- When heated, add the garlic, onion, and jalapeños. Stir-fry for two minutes, scraping the mixture with a metal spatula to keep it moving.
- After adding the chicken, sauté it for two to three minutes, or until the exterior of the flesh starts to brown.
- Add the sugar, soy sauce, basil, and fish sauce and simmer for an additional minute.
- Put on top of rice.

Suck This Advice

Fish sauce, which is made from fermented oily fish, has a strong smell. However, despite its strong aroma, this funky condiment is the foundation of many Southeast Asian cuisines and sauces, giving them a delightfully salty, sweet punch of flavor. Look for a bottle at Asian shops or huge supermarket stores. For those who are new to fish sauce, we feel that the Thai Kitchen brand is the most approachable.

3. Moist Mushroom-Style Chicken

NUTRITION: 270 calories, 420 mg of sodium, and 10 g of fat (3 g saturated).

4 SERVES
You'll need
One tablespoon olive oil, or more if necessary
Four tiny (6 oz each) boneless, skinless chicken breasts
To taste, add salt and black pepper.
minced one medium shallot
8 ounces of sliced cremini mushrooms and 3 chopped garlic cloves
1/4 cup sherry (Sweetheart, fortified wines such as Madeira or Marsala may be used in a pinch.)

1/4 cup dried mushrooms (shiitake, chanterelle, and porcini), steeped for 15 minutes in 1/2 cup warm water

1/2 cup chicken stock reduced in sodium

1⁄ cup of condensed milk

a quarter cup of Greek yogurt

METHODS TO BEGIN

- In a large sauté pan over high heat, heat the olive oil.
- Use salt and black pepper to season the chicken all over.
- When a lovely, deep brown crust forms on the bottom sides of the chicken, add it to the pan and sear it for approximately 3 minutes.
- After 3 minutes, flip the food over and continue cooking until the other side is beautifully browned as well.
- Transfer to a platter.
- Once the chicken has cooked through, add a thin layer of olive oil to the pan.
- When the mushrooms are gently browned, add the shallot, garlic, and

- cremini to the pan and sauté for approximately 3 minutes.
- Put some salt and black pepper over it.
- After adding the sherry, simmer for one minute, scraping up any browned pieces from the pan's bottom with a wooden spoon or spatula.
- Add the half-and-half, chicken stock, and dried mushrooms together with their soaking liquid.
- Lower the heat to a minimum and put the chicken back in the pan.
- Cook the chicken for a further 8 to 10 minutes, or until the liquid has reduced by half and the chicken is well cooked.
- Stir in the yogurt to get a consistent, smooth sauce.
- After dividing the chicken among 4 dishes, drizzle the mushroom sauce over them.

4. Simple Chicken Scaloppine

NOURISHMENT: 280 calories, 11 g fat (3.5 g saturated), 460 mg sodium, and

4 SERVES

You'll need

Four skinless, boneless chicken thighs or breasts (approximately 6 ounces each), uniformly pounded 1 1/4" thick

To taste, add salt and black pepper.

Eight new sage leaves

Four thin prosciutto slices

tsp olive oil

one cup of white wine

1/2 cup chicken stock reduced in sodium

One tablespoon of butter

Raw parsley (may be added).

METHODS TO BEGIN

- Add salt and pepper to the chicken to season it.
- Each breast should have two sage leaves arranged over it. Next, wrap each one with a prosciutto slice, securing the wrap with a toothpick or two.
- In a big skillet, warm the oil over medium heat.
- Once the oil begins to shimmer, place the chicken in it and fry it for 4 to 5 minutes

on each side, or until the chicken is cooked through and firm to the touch, and the prosciutto is crisp and browned.

- Move to four plates.
- When the liquid has reduced by half, add the wine and stock to the pan and simmer, scraping the bottom to release any burned pieces, for approximately two minutes.
- Add a swirl of butter and parsley (if desired).
- After covering the chicken with the sauce, serve.

Consume This Advice.

Some recipes need you to pound the breast of chicken until it becomes a thinner cutlet. The rationale is that meat with a consistent thickness, such as pig, steak, or chicken, cooks more quickly and evenly.

The procedure is simple: Remove the big chopping board and place the chicken on it. Place several layers of plastic wrap over the meat and pound it into submission with a meat mallet or a heavy-based pan.

Of course, cutlets of chicken and other meats are available in many stores, but isn't that kind of boring?

5. Pineapple and Grilled Chicken Sandwich with Spiced Sweet Sauce

NUTRITION: 400 mg of salt, 6 g of fat, and 11 g of calories

4 SERVES
You'll need
4 skinless, boneless chicken breasts weighing 4-6 ounces each
Togarashi sauce
Four Swiss cheese slices
4 ½"-thick pineapple slices
Four wheat buns (Note: A modest amount of whole grains and an excessive amount of sugar

are often used to make whole-wheat buns. Choose a brand that has less than 110 calories and 3 grams of fiber per bun. The best buns in show are Nature's Whitewheat Buns.)
One finely sliced red onion
Pickled red peppers

METHODS TO BEGIN
- Put the chicken in a resealable plastic bag with enough teriyaki sauce to cover it, and marinate it for at least 30 minutes and up to 12 hours in the fridge.
- Turn the grill on high heat. (Holding your hand over the grates should not take more than five seconds.)
- Take the chicken out of the marinade and put it on the grill. Don't throw away any leftover marinade.
- Cook for 4 to 5 minutes on the first side, then turn and top each breast right away with cheese.
- Cook the chicken for a little longer until it is firm to the touch and the cheddar has melted. Take out and put aside.
- Place the pineapple and the buns on the grill while the chicken rests. Cook for

approximately 2 minutes on each side, or until the pineapple is tender and caramelized, and the buns are gently toasted.

- Add pineapple, red onion, jalapeño slices, and chicken on the top of each bun. Brush the chicken with a little extra teriyaki sauce, if you'd like.

Suck This Advice
How to Find Cheaper Chicken at Shops
Although they are the most popular protein in America, boneless, skinless chicken breasts are not the cheapest. Would you want to reduce the sandwich's tab in half? Change to frozen. Men's Health conducted an internal taste test and discovered little to no flavor variation. The only discernible variation? A pound of fresh chicken breast costs around $6, but a pound of frozen chicken breast costs less than $4.

6. Pie au gratin

NUTRITION: 650 mg of sodium, 8 g of saturated fat, and 350 calories

4 SERVES
You'll need
Two tablespoons of butter
One chopped onion, two diced carrots, and two minced garlic cloves
Two cups of cremini or white mushroom stems, and quartered
Two cups of pearl onions, frozen
Two cups of chopped cooked chicken (from a store-bought rotisserie chicken or leftovers)
1½ cups of flour
One cup of whole or 2% milk and two cups of reheated low-sodium chicken broth
1/ cup of cream of tartar
1. Half a cup of frozen peas
To taste, add salt and black pepper.
One sheet of frozen puff pastry
Two egg whites, somewhat whisked

METHODS TO BEGIN

- In a big saucepan or sauté pan, melt the butter over medium heat.
- Once it has melted, add the onion, carrots, and garlic. Cook for approximately 5 minutes, or until the onion is transparent and the carrots start to soften.
- Cook for a further five minutes, stirring often, after adding the pearl onions and mushrooms.
- Using a wooden spoon to ensure that the meat and veggies are equally covered in flour, stir in the chicken and flour.
- Pour the chicken stock in gradually, beating it in with a whisk to prevent the flour from clumping (warm or hot broth helps smooth out the sauce).
- After the stock is mixed in, pour in the milk and half-and-half, cover, and simmer for ten to fifteen minutes, or until the sauce has significantly thickened and is just beginning to stick to the chicken and veggies. Add the peas and mix. Add pepper and salt for seasoning.

- Set oven temperature to 375°F. Divide the pastry into fourths. Using a floured surface, roll out each piece to a 6" square.
- Spoon the chicken mixture into four bowls that can be baked. Using a paring knife, cut off the extra pastry square that covers the top of each bowl. Pinch the dough to seal it around the bowl's edges.
- After brushing the tops with the egg whites, bake for approximately 25 minutes, or until golden brown.

Suck This Advice

The buttery crust that tops the bowls contains the majority of the calories in pot pies. To minimize the calorie effect, this recipe asks for extra thinly rolled puff pastry. However, there are two simple modifications you may use to further limit your consumption of fat:

1) Try using a couple of layers of phyllo dough drizzled with a little butter in place of puff pastry. Even so, compared to puff pastry, it is still lighter and lower in calories.

2) Use an additional 1/2 cup of milk in lieu of the half-and-half.

7. Chipotle-Honey Mustard Oven-Baked
Chicken Fingers.

nutriTION: 350 mg of sodium, 1.5 g of fat (0 g
saturated), and 250 calories.

4 SERVES
You'll need
One pound of skinless, boneless chicken
tenders
To taste, add salt and black pepper.
Three gently beaten egg whites
Two cups gluten-free panko bread crumbs
Two tsp of mustard dijon
1 tsp pure chipotle pepper (This recipe is ideal
for youngsters who like chicken fingers. Simply
make sure the chilies are removed from the
sauce.)
One tablespoon honey

METHODS TO BEGIN
- Set oven temperature to 450°F. Add salt
  and pepper to the chicken to season it.
- The egg whites should be put in a small
  basin. Arrange the crumbs onto a dish
  and further season them.

- After dipping the chicken tenders into the egg, thoroughly coat them with the crumbs.
- After spraying a baking sheet with nonstick cooking spray, place the breaded chicken pieces on it and bake for 10 to 12 minutes, or until the chicken is firm and the crumbs have browned.
- In a large bowl, mix together the mustard, chipotle, and honey.
- Coat each grilled chicken tender equally with the spicy-sweet sauce by tossing them in the mixture.

Suck This Advice

The delicious crunch that comes from a prolonged immersion in sizzling fat is absent from most oven-fried dishes. But replace your bland blue bread crumb canister with these Japanese ones, and you'll have the crispy fried chicken crust without the excess fat. Flat, coarse bread crumbs that may also be gluten-free are called panko. They also provide whatever they coat with a consistently crispy coating. Look for a box in the foreign aisle of your grocery store or order them online.

8. Recipe for Flavor-Boosted, Low-Calorie Chicken Fajitas

NUTRITION: 900 mg of salt, 19 g of fat (3.5 g saturated), and 490 calories

4 SERVES
You'll need
a half-cup of orange juice
Chop 2 tablespoons of chipotle pepper
1 lime's juice
1 teaspoon ground cumin
To taste, add salt and black pepper.
One pound of skinless, boneless chicken breasts
Tbsp canola oil
Eight small (6-inch) flour tortillas, warmed guacamole salsa, and one each of red and green bell peppers and onions sliced
One cup of shredded Cheddar or Jack cheese

METHODS TO BEGIN
- In a sealable plastic bag, combine the orange juice, chipotle, lime juice, cumin, and 1 teaspoon each of salt and pepper.

Add the chicken and let it marinate for an hour in the refrigerator.

- Warm up a grill or grill pan on the stove. Take the chicken out of the marinade and throw away the remaining contents of the bag. The chicken should be cooked through and have a light sear on both sides after 4 to 5 minutes on the grill. Before slicing, let it rest for five minutes.
- Heat the oil in a big cast-iron pan over high heat while the chicken cooks.
- Simmer the onions and bell peppers for ten minutes or until the outsides are caramelized and blackened.
- Add pepper and salt for seasoning.
- Thinly cut the chicken into pieces.
- Bring the pan sizzling to the table with the chicken perched on the hot peppers for a visually striking display.
- Accompany with warm tortillas, salsa, guacamole, and cheese.

Suck This Advice
These four more bases also create excellent fajitas:

Replace the chicken with skirt steak or flank steak marinated in the same sauce.
Peel and devein medium shrimp, then let them marinate in the same marinade for no more than twenty minutes.
Meat Serve Chile Verde with sautéed peppers and onions.
Portobello mushroom caps, either sautéed or grilled and seasoned with chili powder.

9. Alfredo pasta loaded with veggies and chicken.

CALORIES: 540, FAT: 14 g (6 g saturated), SOD: 520 mg

4 SERVES
You'll need
Two tsp unsalted butter
1/4 cup flour
3 mugs 2.2% milk
two chopped garlic cloves
Two tablespoons of finely chopped Parmesan
To taste, add salt and black pepper.

A half-tsp olive oil
Two cups of small broccoli florets
8 ounces of sliced cremini mushrooms
1/4 cup finely diced sun-dried tomato
8 ounces of cooked chicken breast, cut thinly
(rotisserie chicken from the grocery works well
for this)
Whole-wheat fettuccine, 12 ounces

METHODS TO BEGIN
- Melt the butter in a saucepan over medium-low heat to produce the béchamel.
- Add the flour and stir. Simmer for one minute. Stir in the milk gradually so as not to let lumps develop. Add the garlic and boil until pleasantly thickened, stirring often, 10 to 15 minutes.
- Add the Parmesan and salt and pepper to taste. Stay warm.
- In a large skillet or sauté pan, heat the oil over medium-high heat.
- After adding, boil the broccoli for 3 to 4 minutes. Add the tomatoes and mushrooms.

- Simmer the veggies for 5 minutes, or until they start to caramelize slightly.
- Add the chicken and mix. Add pepper and salt for seasoning.
- In the meantime, prepare the pasta as directed on the box.
- After draining, set aside 1 cup of the cooking liquid. Put the pasta back in the saucepan, then toss to coat with the sauce and chicken combination.
- Add a little pasta water to thin down the sauce if it's too thick. Serve right away.

Suck This Advice

That powdery substance you've been shaking for years out of the green can? That isn't Parmigiano. According to Italian government regulations, Parmigiano-Reggiano may only be made from cows that are at least 12 months old and originate from northern Italy. One of the best cheeses in the world is the end product, having a nutty, sweet, and salty taste. On the cheese rind, look for the dotted stamp—this is a reliable indicator of genuineness. Although it's expensive, a $8 chunk can last you for many months.

10. Pasta with Chicken and Spinach

NUTRITION: 9 g fat (3.5 g saturated), 540 mg
salt, and 340 calories

4 SERVES
You'll need
One really big egg
two cups of bread crumbs, panko
1/4 cup of Parmesan cheese, grated
1 teaspoon olive oil
1 tsp of Italian spice
To taste, add salt and black pepper.
Four tiny, skinless, boneless chicken breasts (6
ounces each), each pounded to a consistent
thickness of 1/3 inch
1 12 cups hot tomato sauce, either homemade or
purchased in a jar.
1/2 cup of mozzarella cheese, shredded
Lemon-garlic spinach

METHODS TO BEGIN

- Set oven temperature to 400°F.
- Beat the egg after cracking it into a shallow bowl.
- Mix the bread crumbs, Parmesan, olive oil, Italian seasoning, and a couple of good pinches of salt and black pepper in a different shallow dish (a pie pan works well for this).
- One chicken piece at a time, dip it into the egg, then the bread crumbs, pressing the crumbs into the chicken with your fingertips.
- Arrange the chicken breasts on a roasting pan or baking sheet and put them on the center shelf of the oven.
- Bake for about 12 minutes, or until the bread crumbs are golden brown and the chicken is firm to the touch.
- After taking the chicken out of the oven, turn the oven on broil.
- A generous ladle of tomato sauce and a handful of mozzarella should be spread over each breast. Place the oven rack back in the center position and broil for

about three minutes, or until the cheese is bubbling and melted.

- If desired, top the chicken with more tomato sauce and serve it over the spinach.

11. Baked Chicken With Tomatoes and Capers Inspired by the Med.

NUTRITION: 18 g fat (2.5 g saturated), 420 mg salt, and 310 calories

4 SERVES
You'll need
Four skinless, boneless chicken breasts (4-6 ounces each), uniformly pounded 1 1/4" thick
To taste, add salt and black pepper.
Two cups chopped tomatoes or one pint of cherry tomatoes
1/2 chopped red onion
1/4 cup chopped and pitted green olives
one-fourth cup of pine nuts
Two tablespoons of capers
Two tsp olive oil
Fresh basil, thinly sliced (optional)

METHODS TO BEGIN

- Set oven temperature to 450°F. Add salt and pepper to the chicken to season it.
- To make four trays big enough to fit a chicken breast comfortably, take four large pieces of aluminum foil, fold each in half, and then fold up about 1" of each side. On each piece of foil, place a breast.
- In a mixing dish, combine the tomatoes, onion, olives, pine nuts, capers, and olive oil. Season with a little salt and pepper.
- Place the mixture over the chicken breasts.
- When the chicken is cooked through, place the chicken trays on a baking sheet and bake for approximately 15 minutes. Drizzle the tomato mixture and any remaining foil juices over the dish to serve.
- If using, garnish with basil.

12. Recipe for Chicken Cordon Bleu with Honey Mustard

Nutrition: 12 g fat (6 g saturated), 710 mg sodium, and 350 calories.

4 SERVES
You'll need
Four 6-ounce, skinless, boneless chicken breasts were uniformly crushed. 1 1/4" thick
To taste, add salt and black pepper.
8 slender pieces of salted ham
Four Swiss cheese slices
F2 tablespoons
One beaten egg
1 cup panko breadcrumbs free of gluten (If a gluten-free substitute isn't available, crushed Rice Chex Mix makes a terrific substitute.)
Half a lemon's juice
Two tsp of mustard dijon
One tablespoon honey
A half-tsp olive oil condiment

METHODS TO BEGIN
- Set the oven's temperature to 450 degrees Fahrenheit.

- Use salt and pepper to season the chicken all over.
- Place a pair of ham slices and a single cheese slice on each breast, then gently wrap each one in a wide circular motion to create a compact, jellyroll-esque parcel.
- Put the bread crumbs, egg, and flour into several small dishes.
- Working with one rolled-up breast at a time, gently cover it in flour, then quickly coat it with egg and bread crumbs.
- To ensure that the chicken has an equal coating of crumbs, use your fingers.
- Place the chicken on a baking sheet, cover with the bread crumbs, and bake for 15 to 18 minutes, or until the chicken is cooked through and firm to the touch.
- Mix the mayo, mustard, honey, and lemon juice together to create a smooth, consistent sauce while the chicken bakes.
- Drizzle the honey mustard over the chicken before serving.

Suck This Advice

Breading a chicken
A complete covering of breadcrumbs is necessary for tender, crispy chicken. Almost any pan- or oven-fried dish may be prepared using this technique.

First, pound the chicken until it is 1/4 inch thick while covering it.
Step 2: Dust with flour, then dunk in whipped egg.
Step 3: Use your preferred bread crumbs to completely encase the chicken.

13. Sweet Potato Chicken

NUTRITION: 12 g fat (4.5 g saturated), 480 mg salt, and 330 calories

4 SERVES
You'll need
1/ can (14–16 oz) of drained black beans
1½ teaspoon cumin
1 lime's juice
To taste, add salt and black pepper.

1/2 tablespoon olive or canola oil

Four skinless, boneless (6 oz. apiece) chicken breasts

One cup of ready-made salsa, ideally green (Concocted of tomatillos, onions, jalapeños, and lime, salsa verde perfectly balances acidity and spice, enhancing and enlivening tastes in everything it comes into contact with.)

One cup of pepper jack cheese, shredded

chopped cilantro, fresh

METHODS TO BEGIN

- Set the oven's temperature to 450 degrees Fahrenheit.
- In a saucepan, combine the cumin and black beans and cook thoroughly.
- Add the lime juice and season with salt and pepper to taste.
- Take off the stove, but reheat before serving.
- In a large skillet, heat the oil over medium-high heat.
- Sprinkle the chicken with salt and pepper on both sides, then sear it for three to four minutes on the first side, or until a

- beautiful crust forms, before turning it over.
- After cooking for a further three to four minutes, transfer the meat to the oven with the salsa spooned over it and the cheese on top.
- Bake for no more than five minutes, or until the chicken is well cooked and the cheese is melted and bubbling.
- Arrange the beans onto four plates, add the chicken on top, and sprinkle with the cilantro.

14. Panini with chicken, pesto, and peppers

CALORIES: 450, FAT: 15 g (8 g saturated), SOD 820 mg

4 SERVES
You'll need
Eight pieces of sourdough wholegrain bread
4 tablespoons premade or handmade pesto

4 ounces of thinly sliced fresh mozzarella (fresh mozzarella is more costly than normal mozz but tastes better and has fewer calories). Any kind of shredded part-skim mozzarella would do well in its place, although if you can, try to get some fresh from your neighborhood farmers market.)
34 lb of cooked poultry
one-half cup of roasted peppers
Almond oil

METHODS TO BEGIN

- Turn up the heat to medium in a big cast-iron skillet or stovetop grill pan.
- One spoonful of pesto should be spread over each of the four slices of bread.
- Distribute equal portions of the chicken, red peppers, and mozzarella slices over each piece.
- When the pan is heated, add a thin layer of olive oil and fry the sandwiches (two at a time, if needed) for three to four minutes on each side, or until the cheese has melted and the bread is crispy. (To get optimal results, weigh down the sandwiches with a heavy pan.)

Suck This Advice

A panini maker is a one-trick pony that takes up valuable kitchen storage space, so don't bother spending $100 on it. (In actuality, avoid purchasing any kitchenware with a single use.) Alternatively, consider utilizing a George Foreman grill—millions of Americans already own one—for grilling inside. Just place the sandwich onto the grates that have been warmed (without any oil or butter) and cook it until the inside is melted and the exterior is crispy. Lacking a Foreman? In a pinch, a hot pan works excellent, as does anything hefty to weigh down the sandwich.

15. Pizzaiolo of chicken

NUTRITION: 812 mg of sodium, 369 calories, and 15 g of fat (3 g saturated).

4 SERVES
You'll need
tsp olive oil
Four 6-oz chicken breasts
One teaspoon of dried rosemary or thyme

Add pepper and salt to taste.
Slicing one medium yellow onion and chopping
half a cup of green olives
four minced garlic cloves
1 tsp of chili flakes
28 oz. (one can) mashed up tomatoes
a cup of mozzarella, grated

METHODS TO BEGIN

- Lay the chicken breasts out on a cutting board, cover them with plastic wrap, and pound the chicken into 1/2-inch thick cutlets with a meat mallet or heavy-bottomed pan. Add some thyme or rosemary along with a generous pinch of salt and pepper for seasoning.
- In a large cast-iron skillet or other oven-safe pan, heat the oil over medium-high heat.
- When heated, add the chicken and cook for 3 to 4 minutes, or until the chicken's surface has formed a good crust. Then, turn the chicken and continue cooking for an additional 3 to 4 minutes.
- Take out and set aside the chicken.
- Set the broiler on high.

- Add the garlic, red pepper flakes, onions, and olives to the same pan.
- After around five minutes of sautéing, when the onions have started to softly caramelize, add the tomatoes.
- Return the chicken to the pan after cooking it for an additional three minutes.
- After dividing the mozzarella among the chicken breasts, put the skillet in the oven.
- For three to four minutes, under the broiler, melt and bubble the cheese.
- Spoon enough of the hot red sauce over the chicken before serving.

TURKEY MEALS

1. Sweet Potato Fries with Turkey Meatballs

EACH OF THE 2 SERVING INGREDIENTS
Regarding the meatballs:
1 pound of turkey meat and 1 egg
1/4 tsp of dried oregano
A half-tsp of garlic powder
Tsp of dried basil, half
1 tsp of chili flakes
One teaspoon of salt
Half a cup of fresh parsley, chopped finely
Almond meal, 1/4 cup
Two tsp olive oil

Regarding the sweet potato fries,
4 big, washed and peeled sweet potatoes
Two tsp olive oil
Half a teaspoon of salt

For the sauce to dip cashews:
one head of garlic
Raw cashews, half a cup, soaked for one night,
then drained

two tsp lemon juice
Two tablespoons plus 1/4 cup water

METHODS TO BEGIN
- Set oven temperature to 400°F. Using parchment paper, line two baking sheets.
- The turkey, egg, dried oregano, garlic powder, dried basil, red pepper flakes, salt, minced parsley, and almond meal should all be gently combined in a big bowl. Form golf ball-sized chunks with wet hands, roll them into balls, and place them on a sheet lined with parchment. Give each meatball a quick oil brushing.
- In the meantime, thinly slice the sweet potatoes into 4-inch-long pieces. After putting them on the second baking sheet, cover them with a layer of olive oil and salt. Place the garlic head for the cashew sauce on the baking sheet with the sweet potatoes after wrapping it in foil.
- For 20 to 25 minutes, bake the sweet potatoes and meatballs. Slice through one meatball to ensure it is cooked all the way through. Take the meatballs out of the oven if that's the case. Continue baking

the sweet potatoes for another 10 to 15 minutes, or until they're crispy, turning them over once halfway through.

- Once the potatoes are done, remove from oven and carefully unwrap the garlic from the foil. Let cool slightly until cool enough to handle.
- Squeeze the roasted garlic cloves from their skins and place them in a blender with the cashews, lemon juice, and water. Blend until smooth and creamy.
- Serve the meatballs with the sweet potato fries and dipping sauce on the side.

2. Turkey Bolognese With Fettuccine.

NUTRITION: 520 calories, 10 g fat (2.5 g saturated), 520 mg sodium

SERVES 4
YOU'LL NEED
½ Tbsp olive oil
1 small onion, diced
2 stalks celery, diced 1 medium carrot, peeled and diced
2 cloves garlic, minced
8 ounces ground white turkey 8 oz ground sirloin
1 link Italian-style turkey sausage, casing removed
1 cup dry white wine
½ cup 2% milk
½ cup low-sodium chicken stock
1 can (28 oz) smashed tomatoes
2 Tbsp tomato paste
1 bay leaf
Salt and black pepper to taste
1 packet (12 ounces) fresh fettuccine or 8 oz dried egg noodles
Finely grated Parmesan for serving

METHODS TO BEGIN

- Heat the olive oil in a big saucepan over medium heat.
- Add the onion, celery, carrot, and garlic and sauté for 5 minutes, until softened.
- Add the ground turkey, sirloin, and sausage, using a wooden spoon to break the meat into tiny pieces.
- Simmer the beef for about 7 minutes, or until it is well cooked.
- Stir in the tomatoes, tomato paste, wine, milk, and bay leaf.
- Reduce the heat to low and simmer the sauce over very low heat for at least 45 minutes, but ideally up to 90 minutes.
- Use salt and pepper to season to taste. Throw away the bay leaf.
- Cook the pasta in boiling salted water for 3 to 4 minutes, or until it's just al dente.
- Empty and put back into the pot.
- Place on the burner over very low heat, then slowly add a few large spoonfuls of the Bolognese sauce at a time, stirring to ensure the noodles are well coated.

- You should use around two-thirds of the sauce you make, as you will have plenty for the pasta.
- The spaghetti should be divided among 4 heated bowls or plates.
- At the table, pass the Parmesan.

Suck This Advice

The sauce from the Bolognese recipe is more than enough for this dish, which is intentional as it tastes even better the following day. Here are some ideas for using the leftovers.

Put on top of soft polenta.

Layer the turkey Bolognese, Parmesan, and béchamel over no-bake noodles to make one heck of a lasagna.

Stuff inside a toasted bread, a la sloppy Joe from Italy.

3. Turkey meatballs and lean spaghetti

NUTRITION: 740 mg of sodium, 12.5 g of fat (5 g saturated), and 510 calories

4 SERVES

You'll need

Two pieces of bread soaked in five minutes of milk

12 ounces of turkey breast meat

Ground beef, 12 oz, 85% lean

1/2 cup chopped parsley and one egg, with more for garnish

Add extra Parmesan cheese for garnish (two tablespoons)

1/4 tsp salt, 1/2 tsp pepper, and 1 chopped onion

three minced garlic cloves

Two tsp olive oil

28 oz. (one can) whole tomatoes with peels (we adore Muir Glen)

DeCecco Whole Wheat Spaghetti, one pound

METHODS TO BEGIN

- Tear the bread into small pieces after taking it out of the milk and squeezing off most of the liquid.
- Combine the meat, turkey, egg, Parmesan, parsley, salt, pepper, and half

of the onion and garlic. Shape into golf ball-sized spheres.

- In a large nonstick skillet or sauté pan, heat half the olive oil and cook the meatballs over medium heat until nicely browned. Put away.
- The remaining onion and garlic should be cooked over medium heat in a skillet with the remaining tablespoon of olive oil until they become transparent.
- Simmer after adding the tomatoes.
- Cook the meatballs for 15 to 20 minutes after adding them.
- Pasta should be cooked as directed on the box until it is al dente.
- Distribute it among six dishes or plates, add the meatballs and sauce on top, then sprinkle the Parmesan and parsley on top.

Consume This Money-Saving Strategy

You think the secret to a superb pasta sauce is using fresh tomatoes? Rethink it. They may cost up to three times as much as canned tomatoes, cost more to prepare, and have unpredictable effects (particularly in the winter when tomatoes are imported from the southern hemisphere). When tomato season is at its peak, tomatoes are gathered and canned right away. Your best option is to use whole peeled tomatoes since they have undergone the least amount of processing and have the strongest tomato taste.

4. Healthy Recipe for 7-Layer Dip

NUTRITION: 480 mg of salt, 13 g of fat (2 g saturated), and 280 calories

SERVES 6
Requirement:
Ten corn tortillas, divided into triangular shapes
Tbsp canola oil
Add salt to taste.
1 teaspoon olive oil

1 tsp chile powder and 8 oz ground turkey

1/4 teaspoon cayenne

to taste, black pepper

One can (15 oz) of rinsed and drained black beans

1 lime's juice

1-tsp cumin

1/4 cup guacamole or premade guacamole

One 4-oz can roasted green chilies, chopped

1/2 cup store-bought salsa or pico de gallo

1/4 cup Greek yogurt with 2%

1/2 cup black olives, cut or sliced

METHODS TO BEGIN

- Turn the oven on to 425°F. After tossing the tortillas in the canola oil, arrange them on a baking sheet. (To prevent the chips from overlapping, you may need to use two sheets.)
- Bake until crispy and golden brown, approximately 10 minutes. After they are taken out of the oven, sprinkle with salt.
- In a medium sauté pan, heat the olive oil over medium heat while the tortillas are baking.

- Season the turkey with salt, pepper, chili powder, and cayenne as it cooks, and simmer for approximately five minutes, until it is cooked through.
- Add the cumin, lime juice, salt, and black pepper to taste, and mix the black beans.
- Build the dip in a large glass serving dish or ramekin: Line the bottom with guacamole, then cover with black beans, turkey, chiles, pico de gallo, yogurt, and olives.
- Present beside the tortilla chips.

5. Low-Carb Sausage

The majority of breakfast sausages include some sweetness, usually from brown sugar or maple syrup. Obviously, they aren't quite Paleo, so this dish goes in a different direction. Add a teaspoon of coconut sugar and diced Gala or Honeycrisp apples to the sausage to make it sweeter. These very sweet and flowery apple cultivars will prevent the taste of this sausage from getting too monotonous.

TEN PATTIES EACH INGREDIENT
One teaspoon each of fennel and cumin seeds
One pound of ground chicken or turkey
Four garlic cloves, crushed and cut coarsely
One medium-sized Honeycrisp or Gala apple cut finely
One teaspoon of coconut sugar
Two tsp kosher salt
Half a teaspoon of freshly ground pepper
Optional: 1/4 teaspoon crushed red pepper
One or two tablespoons of olive oil

METHODS TO BEGIN
- Add the cumin and fennel seeds to a pan and cook over medium-low heat. Cook for three to five minutes, stirring often, or until spices are aromatic. To cool, move the spices to a dish.
- Using your hands, thoroughly incorporate the cooled fennel and cumin seeds, turkey or chicken, garlic, apple,

coconut sugar, salt, black pepper, and red pepper, if desired, in a large bowl.

- Make 10 identical patties out of the mixture, each approximately ½ inch thick. If patties won't be cooked right away, freeze them for an hour on a sheet pan coated with foil or parchment paper, then move them to freezer bags.
- One tablespoon of oil should be heated over medium heat in a large nonstick or cast-iron pan if cooking right away. Grease the pan with extra oil and fry the patties in two batches, cooking them for 5 minutes on each side, or until the beef reaches an internal temperature of 165 ºF.

6. Sloppy Joe Recipe for Turkey

NUTRITION: 820 mg of sodium, 11 g of fat (2.5 g saturated), and 340 calories

4 SERVES
You'll need

A half-tsp olive oil
One big onion, chopped
One chopped green bell pepper
1.5 cups tomato sauce and one pound of lean ground turkey
Double-stick tomato paste
Two tsp of brown sugar
One tablespoon of red wine vinegar
One tablespoon of Worcestershire sauce
A half-tsp of chili powder
Tabasco or other spicy sauce in ten to twelve shakes
To taste, add salt and black pepper.
Four toasted whole-wheat or sesame rolls

METHODS TO BEGIN

- In a large skillet or sauté pan, heat the oil over medium heat.
- When the onion and bell pepper are softened, sauté them for approximately two minutes.
- When the turkey is just browned, add it and continue to cook, breaking up the flesh with a wooden spoon.
- Salt and pepper should be added along with tomato sauce, tomato paste, sugar,

vinegar, Worcestershire, chili powder, and spicy sauce.
- Reduce the heat to a minimum. Simmer until the liquid has reduced and the meat is well coated in sauce, about 10 minutes.
- Spoon mixture onto each roll.

Suck This Advice

Ground chicken or lean sirloin works as well in place of turkey in this recipe. It may seem absurd, but a couple of fillets of finely diced catfish perform really well as a healthier substitute, and they taste amazing too. In addition, it's a great way to get a small amount of fish in your diet.

Remember to stock up on napkins since this delicious dish will be just as messy as the traditional version, regardless of the meat you pick.

7. A hearty, low-fat recipe for turkey chili

NUTRITION: 490 mg of sodium, 6 g of fat (1 g saturated), and 330 calories

SERVES 6
REQUIREMENT
One tablespoon of canola
One big onion, diced; two minced garlic cloves
1 teaspoon ground cumin
1½ teaspoon of dried oregano
1/4 cup powdered chilis
1½ teaspoon of ground cinnamon
Two bay leaves.
Lean ground turkey, 2 pounds
Double-stick tomato paste
1 oz (1 piece) dark chocolate or 1 tablespoon powdered cocoa
One 12-ounce bottle or can of ale
Chop 1 tablespoon of chipotle pepper
28 oz. (one can) entire tomatoes with peels
One can (14.2 oz) of rinsed and drained white beans
One can (14.2 oz) of rinsed and drained pinto beans
To taste, add salt and black pepper.

To taste, add cayenne or hot sauce (optional).
Lime wedges, shredded cheese, chopped scallions, raw onions, and optional sour cream

METHODS TO BEGIN

- In a big saucepan, warm the oil over medium heat. Add the onion and garlic, and simmer for approximately 5 minutes, or until the onion becomes transparent.
- Cook for a further two to three minutes, or until the spices are quite aromatic, after adding the cumin, oregano, chili powder, cinnamon, and bay leaves.
- When the turkey is no longer pink, add the tomato paste and mix with a wooden spoon.
- Incorporate the beer, cocoa, chipotle, and tomatoes, ensuring that each tomato is somewhat chunky but not entire by pressing it between your fingers.
- After lowering the heat, simmer for forty-five minutes.
- After adding the beans, season with pepper and salt.

- Taste and add your preferred spicy sauce or a couple of pinches of cayenne if you want your chili hotter.
- Bring the beans to a boil. Garnish with your preferred toppings and serve.

Suck This Advice

The spices are what distinguish competitive chili chefs from one another, not the meat or beans (almost all of them use chuck and onions and nothing else). In a pinch, premade chili powder works very well, although fresh is always preferable. Anchos are fruity and mild, New Mexican chiles are earthy, and chiles de arbol are scorching hot. Purchase a variety of dried chiles from a Mexican grocery store, remove the stems and seeds, roast the peppers for a short while on a dry pan, and then crush the peppers into a powder in a coffee grinder. You may count on your next batch to be of competitive standard.

8.   Meatloaf with Turkey

NUTRITION: 920 mg of sodium, 11 g of fat (3 g saturated), and 290 calories

SERVES 4 ARE NEEDED
About the meatloaf of turkey:
1 little onion, cut into quarters and peeled
Quartered and stemmed one-and-a-half red bell pepper
One little carrot, peeled and coarsely sliced
two peeled garlic cloves
1 1/2 pounds of turkey meat
a half-cup of breadcrumbs
1/4 cup chicken stock with minimal sodium
One beaten egg
Worcestershire, 1 teaspoon
One teaspoon of low-sodium soy sauce
A half-tsp of dried thyme
1/2 tsp each of salt and black pepper

To make the glaze:
1½ cups of ketchup
Two tsp of brown sugar
Two tsp of soy sauce (low sodium)

Two tsp of vinegar from apple cider

METHODS TO BEGIN

- Set oven temperature to 325°F.
- In a food processor, combine the onion, bell pepper, carrot, and garlic; pulse until finely chopped. (If a food processor isn't available, you may do this by hand.)
- In a large mixing bowl, combine the veggies with the turkey, bread crumbs, Worcestershire, soy sauce, and egg, and season with salt and black pepper.
- Till the ingredients are all dispersed equally, gently stir.
- Pour the meatloaf mixture into a 13" x 9" baking dish, then shape the loaf into an approximately 9" long by 6" broad loaf with your hands.
- Combine the glaze ingredients and brush the mixture over the meatloaf.
- Bake for one hour, or until an instant-read thermometer put into the middle of the loaf registers 160°F and the glaze has become a rich shade of crimson.

Suck This Advice

The finest option, in our opinion, is still a thick meatloaf sandwich, but there are plenty of ways to reimagine meatloaf the following day—for example, by covering it with sautéed peppers and onions or topping it with a fried egg. While the meatloaf reheats at 325°F, gently sauté onions until well caramelized. Top with a thin slice of smoked gouda and serve the whole dish on a toasted bun. Just the sandwich alone makes this dish worthwhile.

9. Southwest Turkey Burger

Nutrition: 470 calories, 26 g fat (7 g saturated), 520 mg salt.

4 SERVES
You'll need
Two tsp olive oil mayo
1 tablespoon pure chipotle
Thumbful of lime juice
1 pound of turkey meat

One tablespoon of Magic Blackening Rub (one tablespoon each of paprika, salt, black pepper, ground cumin, garlic powder, onion powder, dried oregano, and ½ tsp cayenne pepper)
To taste, add salt and black pepper.
4 pepper slices Monterey Jack or Jack cheese
Four gently toasted English muffins or potato rolls
One avocado, finely cut, pitted and peeled
1/2 cup prepared or store-bought pico de gallo

METHODS TO BEGIN
- Mix the lime juice, chipotle puree, and mayo in a mixing bowl. Hold back.
- Heat a cast-iron skillet, grill pan, or barbecue to a medium temperature.
- Shape the turkey into four equal patties with gentle pressure, taking care not to overwork the flesh as this might result in tough, thick burgers.
- In addition to salt and black pepper, season the burgers on both sides with the blackening rub.
- Grill the burgers for about 4 minutes, or until the bottoms have developed a beautiful, brown crust.

- Turn over and cover with cheese right away.
- Cook for a further 4 minutes or so, or until the burger is barely firm to the touch and the cheese has melted.
- After layering the avocado slices and Pico de Gallo on top of four English muffin halves, top each with a burger.
- After topping the burgers with chipotle mayo, serve.

Suck This Advice
Since turkey is a lean meat, substituting it for beef in burgers is a very beneficial move. When selecting the brand of meat to purchase, use additional attention to ensure that it's a healthy decision. Choose products from companies that stand true to their name—Applegate Naturals—by avoiding artificial ingredients.

10. Recipe for Cheesy Turkey Meatloaf Muffins

NUTRITION: 16 g fat (8 g saturated), 985 mg salt, and 334 calories

PAIRS SIX GUNNERS

Components

Greaseless cooking spray

1 1/2 pounds ground turkey, divided into 1/4
cup of ketchup

one cup of cheddar cheese, grated

one cup of finely chopped onion

One cup of standard panko bread crumbs

1/4 cup milk, 2%

One gently beaten egg

Two tsp of sauce Worcestershire

two minced garlic cloves

1/4 teaspoon poultry spice

One teaspoon of salt

half a teaspoon of ground pepper

METHODS TO BEGIN

- Turn the oven on to 350°F. Apply nonstick cooking spray to six regular muffin cups and put them aside.
- In a large bowl, add ground turkey, cheese, onion, bread crumbs, Worcestershire sauce, garlic, poultry seasoning, salt, and pepper. Mix well to fully blend.

- Distribute the mixture among the six muffin tins that have been prepared, spreading them equally, pushing down lightly, and then piling the tops.
- Apply the remaining 1/4 cup of ketchup on top. Bake for about 45 minutes, or until an instant-read thermometer reads 170°F internally.
- Before serving, let it sit for five minutes.

11. Fish tacos with avocado and spicy tuna

NUTRITION: 330 calories, 460 mg of salt, and 13 g of fat (2 g saturated).

4 SERVES
You'll need
Four cups of green or red cabbage shredded
Two tsp olive oil mayo
One lime's juice and lime wedges for serving
1/2 tsp of chipotle pepper, canned
To taste, add salt and black pepper.
1/2 tablespoon olive or canola oil
12 ounces of fresh ahi or premium tuna

8 tortillas de maiz
One mature avocado, cut, pitted, and peeled
Relish pickled onions
fiery sauce

METHODS TO BEGIN
- In a large mixing bowl, combine the cabbage, mayo, chipotle, and lime juice.
- Add pepper and salt for seasoning. Put the slaw on hold. (To enable the flavors to marry, it's ideal to do this at least 15 minutes before cooking.)
- In a big cast-iron skillet or sauté pan made of stainless steel, heat the oil over medium-high heat.
- Use a generous amount of black pepper and salt to season the tuna.
- When the oil is heated, add the tuna and sear it for two minutes on each side, or until the interior of the fish is still rare despite the development of a lovely crust.
- Heat the tortillas in the pan until the outsides are just beginning to crisp up.
- Cut the tuna into thin pieces.

- Spoon into each tortilla, then garnish with pickled onions, slaw, and avocado slices.
- Accompany with spicy sauce and lime wedges.

Suck This Advice

Soaking in a pickle brine gives veggies like onions, cucumbers, and peppers the ideal vinegar bite. Mix equal quantities of rice wine vinegar or apple cider vinegar with a generous pinch of salt and sugar. Mix everything together and add the veggies. Let it sit for a minimum of 10 minutes before serving with your fish tacos. They may be refrigerated for up to a week when covered.

12. Cornmeal Catfish in the Style of the South with Tomato Gravy

NUTRITION: 500 mg of salt, 16 g of fat (3.5 g saturated), and 340 calories

4 SERVES
You'll need
Two tablespoons of rendered bacon fat
12 cups + 2 Tbsp of ground cornmeal
one can (14.5" oz) entire tomatoes with peels
on, gently mashed, and fluids thrown out
To taste, add salt and black pepper.
Tbsp canola oil
1/8 teaspoon cayenne
Four 6-ounce fillets of catfish

METHODS TO BEGIN

- In a medium saucepan, melt the bacon grease over low heat.
- When the cornmeal is light golden, add the remaining 2 tablespoons and cook, stirring frequently, for approximately 5 minutes.
- Simmer for a further ten minutes after adding the drained tomatoes. Put some salt and black pepper over it.
- As the sauce is simmering, get the catfish ready. In a large cast-iron skillet or nonstick pan, heat the oil over medium heat.

- In a shallow dish, spread out the ½ cup of cornmeal and add a large teaspoon of salt and black pepper along with the cayenne.
- After giving the catfish a cornmeal dusting on both sides, put it in the heated pan.
- Fry for 6 to 8 minutes, rotating once, or until the fish flakes easily with a little touch of your finger and the top is golden brown and crusty.
- Place a generous portion of tomato gravy on top of each fillet.

13. Sandwich with blackened fish with cabbage and avocado.

NUTRITION: 460 calories, 620 mg of salt, and 14 g of fat (2.5 g saturated).

4 SERVES
You'll need
One cup of simple Greek yogurt

One tsp Sriracha Lime juice
Tbsp canola oil
Four fillets of catfish or tilapia (6 oz each)
1 tablespoon spice (blackening)
4 whole-wheat buns with sesame seeds
One pitted, peeled, and sliced avocado
Two cups of red cabbage, shredded
Salted onions

METHODS TO BEGIN
- Mix the lime juice, sriracha, and yogurt together. Put away.
- In a large cast-iron skillet, heat the oil over high heat. Season the fish fillets with a generous amount of blackening spice on both sides.
- Once the pan's oil begins to smoke, add the fish and cook it for three minutes without moving, until a brown crust develops.
- After flipping the fillets, heat for a further two to three minutes, or until your fingertip can easily flake the fish.
- Toast the buns under the broiler, cut side up, while the fish cooks. Spoon the cabbage and avocado onto each bun. Add

the onions, yogurt sauce, and hot fish over top.

Suck This Advice

One of our favorite cooking methods is blackening, not just because it tastes so good, but also because the strong spice rub covers anything it comes into contact with and leaves a powerful antioxidant coating. You may use this cooking method on a number of meats by following these three easy stages for pork, chicken, or fish.

Step 1: Apply about 1/4 tsp of blackening seasoning on both sides of each piece of fish or meat.
Step 2: Cook in a very hot, canola oil-coated cast-iron pan without stirring, until a brown crust forms.
Step 3: Cook through by flipping and repeating.

14. Swordfish grilled with caponata

NUTRITION: 520 mg of sodium, 11 g of fat (2.5 g saturated), and 360 calories

4 SERVES
You'll need
One tablespoon of olive oil, plus more for the fish's coating; two medium eggplants, chopped into ⁄2" cubes
Diced one medium onion
two minced garlic cloves
One can (14.2 oz) cut-up tomatoes
Two tablespoons of raisins, ideally golden ones
Two tablespoons of capers
One tablespoon of red wine vinegar
1 teaspoon sugar
1/4 cup of freshly chopped basil
To taste, add salt and black pepper.
4 little, 6-ounce swordfish steaks

METHODS TO BEGIN

- In a medium saucepan set over medium heat, warm the olive oil.
- Add the eggplant, onion, and garlic; sauté until softened and lightly browned, approximately 5 minutes.
- Stir in the sugar, vinegar, capers, raisins, and tomatoes.
- Once the veggies are extremely soft and the mixture has the consistency of

marmalade, cover and boil for 15 minutes.

- Add the basil and season with black pepper and salt. Stay warm.
- Turn the heat up to medium-high on a grill or grill pan.
- Swordfish should be seasoned with salt and black pepper on both sides after being coated in olive oil. Cook the steaks for 4 minutes, or until attractive grill marks appear. If you'd like, you may turn the steaks over halfway through to get diamond-shaped grill marks.
- After flipping, cook for a further 4 minutes or until your fingertip can easily pierce the skin.
- Spoon plenty of caponata over the top of each swordfish plate.
- This dish is derived from one of our Cook This, Not That! books, along with hundreds more. You may also purchase the book for more simple cooking ideas!

15. Healthful Grilled Swordfish Steak with Pesto Topper

nutriTION: 390 mg of sodium, 13 g of fat (3 g saturated), and 250 calories

4 SERVES
You'll need
Two tsp bottled pesto
Four steaks of swordfish (4-6 ounces each)
1 tablespoon olive oil
Two peeled and slightly smashed garlic cloves
two cups of sweet cherries
To taste, add salt and black pepper.

METHODS TO BEGIN
- After applying the pesto all over the swordfish steaks, cover them and let them marinate for half an hour in the refrigerator.
- In a sauté pan set over medium heat, warm the olive oil while the fish marinates.
- When the garlic is just browned, add it and simmer for one or two minutes.

- Add the tomatoes and sauté for approximately 5 minutes, or until the skins are gently blistered and ready to burst.
- Add pepper and salt for seasoning.
- Set a grill or grill pan to preheat.
- Use salt and pepper to season the fish all over.
- Once the grill is hot, cook the swordfish for 4 to 5 minutes on each side, or until the flesh flakes easily with light pressure and the fish is cooked through.
- Warm up the tomatoes and place a spoonful on top of each steak.
- Suck This Advice
- Increased Preferences for Grains and Pesto
- Every home-cooked meal in America must include some kind of starch, generally rice or potatoes, both of which are nothing more than empty carbohydrates. However, a brand-new class of whole grains that may reduce calories and increase nutrients has inundated the market. We really like the South American quinoa, but you should

also try amaranth, couscous, bulgar, and farro. These are all great high-fiber substitutes for potatoes and rice.

-

- And let's discuss the many pesto options while we're at it! Enjoy the change? Basil, pine nuts, and parmesan cheese form the foundation of traditional pesto, but there are many more delicious combinations as well. Trader Joe's Kale Cashew Pesto is what we suggest. It's vegan as well as relish!

16. Broccoli with Shrimp in an Instant Pot

Components
1 pound of fresh or frozen shrimp
2 crowns of broccoli
1/4 cup sesame oil
two minced cloves of garlic
Two tsp freshly grated ginger
Two tsp of oyster sauce
One teaspoon of brown sugar
One tablespoon of rice wine vinegar
Seeds of semen

Green onion with Sriracha

METHODS TO BEGIN
- Trim and chop the broccoli crowns into smaller pieces.
- Use clean hands to deshell any fresh shrimp you purchase. Make careful to defrost them in the refrigerator overnight if you purchased them frozen. Additionally, deshell them if necessary.
- Combine the oyster sauce, brown sugar, rice wine vinegar, soy sauce, ginger, and chopped garlic in the Instant Pot. Mix by whisking.
- Put the shrimp and broccoli into the Instant Pot. After sealing the Instant Pot, cook it for one minute at high pressure (Manual or Pressure Cook).
- Release the pressure as soon as the buzzer sounds.
- Serve the shrimp and broccoli with sesame seeds, chopped green onion, and sriracha on top of rice (or cauliflower rice if you're trying to make it low-carb).

17. Fish Bowl Tacos

EACH OF THE 2 SERVING INGREDIENTS
About the fish:
Two tsp olive oil
two salmon filets, medium
1½ teaspoon cumin
1/4 tsp powdered garlic
Add pepper and salt.

Regarding the avocado:
One juicy avocado
Diced half a tiny red onion
Chop 1 tablespoon of cilantro.
1/2 lime juice
Sea salt 1/4 tsp cumin

For the salsa de mango:
One ripe mango cut up
½ teaspoon sea salt
½ teaspoon olive oil
1/2 lime juice

About the slaw
Half a head of finely sliced cabbage
Two medium carrots, thinly sliced
1 teaspoon olive oil
A half-tsp of white vinegar
One-fourth teaspoon salt

Regarding the riced cauliflower:
tsp olive oil
One big head of cauliflower, cored and coarsely chopped
Two tsp of coconut milk
Add pepper and salt.

METHODS TO BEGIN
- To prepare the salmon, place a large pan over medium heat and add enough oil to get it hot but not smoking. On both sides of the salmon, evenly distribute the

cumin, garlic powder, salt, and pepper. When the fish is cooked through, add it to the pan and cook for approximately 4 minutes. Then, turn it over and cook for an additional 2 to 3 minutes. Place on a platter.

- To prepare the guacamole: Mash the avocado and mix in the onion, cilantro, lime juice, cumin, and salt in a small bowl. Toss to blend thoroughly. Place plastic wrap over it and leave it there.

- Toss the mango with the olive oil, lime juice, and salt in a small dish to make the mango salsa. Put away.

- To make the slaw, mix the cabbage, carrots, oil, vinegar, and salt in a medium bowl. Toss to mix, then put aside.

- To prepare the cauliflower rice, heat the oil in a large pan over medium heat until it is hot but not smoking. Add the coconut milk and cauliflower, then season with the salt and pepper. Cook the cauliflower for 5 to 8 minutes over medium-high heat, stirring periodically, until it softens.

- Create the bowls: After dividing the cauliflower rice between two bowls, evenly distribute the guacamole, mango salsa, and slaw on top. Place a salmon filet on top of each.

18. Fry Coconut Shrimp in the Air

SERVES FOUR PIECES
Half a cup of shredded coconut without sugar
1/4 cup of coconut milk in a can
half a cup of Panko
One pound of medium shrimp, cooked, skinned, and deveined
Fourth and Heart Cooking Spray, or any other cooking spray for high heat
Add pepper and salt to taste.

METHODS TO BEGIN
- Toast the coconut for a few minutes over low heat in a small pan until golden brown.
- Pour the coconut milk into a small bowl. Put the toasted coconut and Panko into another shallow dish and stir.

- After using a paper towel to pat dry, dip the shrimp into the coconut milk and then the Panko mixture.
- Set the air fryer's temperature to 400°F. Working in batches if necessary, place the shrimp in the air fryer in a single layer. Fry until golden brown, approximately 7 minutes, rotating halfway through. Add pepper and salt for seasoning.

19. Recipe for Low-Calorie Baked Fish and Chips

NUTRITION: 810 mg of sodium, 14 g of fat (1.5 g saturated), and 380 calories

4 SERVES
You'll need
4 six-ounce cod fillets each
1 cup buttermilk without fat
Taste of Tabasco
one-fourth cup of panko bread crumbs
1/4 cup of chips with crushed salt and vinegar
To taste, add salt and black pepper.

Two tsp olive oil condiment
Two tsp of Greek yogurt
lime juice from one
Chop 2 tablespoons of pickles
One tablespoon of capers
1 teaspoon Dijon mustard

METHODS TO BEGIN

- Put the fish, buttermilk, and several shakes of Tabasco into a plastic bag that can be sealed. Let it marinate for 20 minutes in the fridge.
- Set oven temperature to 400°F.
- In a shallow baking dish, combine the bread crumbs and smashed chips. Season with a couple pinches of salt and black pepper.
- Fish should be taken out of the buttermilk one piece at a time and rolled in the coating. Use your fingers to massage the coating over the fish's surface.
- The breaded fish should be placed on a rack inside a baking sheet. Bake for about 15 minutes, or until the fish flakes easily with a finger pressed gently and the

coating is attractively browned and crispy.

- In a mixing bowl, combine the yogurt, mayo, pickles, capers, lemon juice, and Dijon while the fish bakes.
- A dollop of tartar sauce should be served beside the fish.

20. Crispy Quesadilla with Chipotle Shrimp

ENERGY: 340 calories, 8 g saturated fat, 15 g fat, and 750 mg sodium

4 SERVES
You'll need
Peel and deveined 8 oz. medium shrimp
a half-cup of orange juice
1 tablespoon chipotle pepper from a can
two minced garlic cloves
A half-tsp canola oil
One medium onion chopped One bell pepper, either red or yellow, chopped
To taste, add salt and black pepper.
Four substantial whole-wheat tortillas

Two cups of Monterey Jack cheese, shredded
Avocado Salsa

METHODS TO BEGIN

- Add the chipotle pepper, garlic, and orange juice to the shrimp. For 15 minutes, marinate.
- In a big cast-iron skillet or sauté pan, heat the oil over medium-high heat.
- Add the onion and pepper and simmer for approximately 10 minutes, or until the outside is gently browned and the oil is just beginning to smoke.
- Place the shrimp in the middle of the pan and push the veggies to the sides.
- Sauté for ten minutes or until the food is cooked thoroughly.
- To taste, add salt and pepper for seasoning. Take off the heat source.
- Apply cooking spray, oil, or butter to a different nonstick pan and place it over medium-low heat. Lay a tortilla on the bottom, cover with half of the cheese, then add another tortilla on top and cover with the remaining half of the shrimp mixture.

- Cook until the bottom is very crisp, approximately 5 minutes. Then, turn and continue cooking for an additional 2 to 3 minutes.
- Scoop out the quesadillas and, if desired, top with guacamole and salsa.

Suck This Advice

Desire a crunchy quesadilla? The ideal way to cook quesadillas is to cook them on a cast-iron or non-stick pan, but this isn't the only way to do it. Do you have a large quantity? Preheat the grill and cook them directly on the well-oiled grates for a few minutes on each side. Alternatively, bake them for 12 minutes at 450 ∨F, turning them once during that time.

21. Blackened Tilapia with Garlic-Lime Butter

Nutritional Information: 300 calories, 14 g fat (6 g saturated), 510 mg sodium.

4 SERVES

You'll need

Two tablespoons of softened room-temperature butter

Tbsp finely chopped, fresh cilantro

Two garlic cloves, finely chopped

One teaspoon of lime zest and one lime's juice

Tbsp canola oil

Four fillets of tilapia (6 oz apiece)

One teaspoon of Magic Blackening Rub

METHODS TO BEGIN

- In a small mixing bowl, combine the butter, cilantro, garlic, lime zest, and lime juice; swirl to fully combine. Put away.

- In a large cast-iron skillet or sauté pan, heat the oil over high heat. Apply the blackening rub all over the fish.

- As soon as the oil in the pan begins to slightly smoke, add the fish and cook it for 3 to 4 minutes on the first side, without moving, until the spice rub becomes crusty and black.

- After flipping, cook for another minute or two, or until your fingertip can easily flake the fillets.

- After transferring the fish to four serving dishes, drizzle a little of the flavored butter over each one right away.

Suck This Advice

The Expert Method: Darkening

Using a cast-iron skillet that is very hot is the best approach to get the desired complete sear. Apply a thin layer of oil to the skillet and heat it to the maximum temperature (also turn on the kitchen fan). The fish or meat should be added carefully after you see smoke rising from the oil in little puffs. You want a black crust to form over the protein, and fumbling with the food will stop that from occurring. Leave it alone for at least two minutes. Cook on one side for 75% of the cooking time, then turn and continue cooking on the other side.

22.   Tilapia with Vegetables in the Instant Pot

EACH OF THE 2 SERVING INGREDIENTS

2 new fillets of tilapia

One cup of chopped carrots

One cup of green peas
one-fourth cup of vegetable broth
One tablespoon of butter
Parsley for decoration
freshly split pepper

METHODS TO BEGIN

- Place the green beans and carrots in the bottom of the Instant Pot.
- Place the two fillets of tilapia on top of the trivet.
- Cover the fish with the veggie broth. Cut the butter into cubes and add them to the fish.
- Put the cover on and cook for 8 minutes on high pressure (Manual or Pressure Cook). Release the pressure as soon as the Instant Pot beeps.
- Before serving, garnish the fish with freshly cracked pepper and parsley.

23. Melt of Italian tuna.

NUTRITION: 980 mg of sodium, 13 g of fat (2 g saturated), and 340 calories

4 SERVES
You'll need
Two 5-ounce cans each the drained tuna
One little red onion, chopped
1/4 cup finely diced green olives
Two tsp olive oil condiment
Two tsp bottled pesto
1 tablespoon minced and washed capers
lime juice from one
Eight pieces of wheat bread
Two ounces of freshly sliced mozzarella (you may also use low-fat shredded mozzarella)
One big chopped tomato
Roughly 1 teaspoon olive oil

METHODS TO BEGIN

- Tuna, onion, olives, mayo, pesto, capers, and lemon juice should all be combined in a mixing bowl and stirred.
- Heat a nonstick or cast-iron pan to a medium temperature.
- Spread a small amount of olive oil on both sides of the sandwiches, then heat for 2 to 3 minutes on each side, or until

the cheese has melted and the bread is toasted.

Suck This Advice

One of the largest misnomers in the food industry is "tuna salad." While both "tuna" and "salad" are healthful when eaten separately, they cause problems when mixed. Resurrect this problematic duo with some more astute combinations from your spice cabinet:

Golden raisins, cashews, curry powder, and shredded carrot

Jack cheese, avocado slices, and salsa

Sun-dried tomatoes, provolone, and artichokes.

24.   Keto Avocado-Blueberry Salsa paired with Seared Ginger-Cumin Swordfish

NUTRITION: 35 g protein, 6 g fiber, 3 g sugar, 4 g saturated fat, 536 mg sodium, and 392 calories.

EACH OF THE 2 SERVING INGREDIENTS

For the swordfish, cut two 6-ounce, 3/4-inch-thick swordfish fillets.

two tsp lime juice

1 tsp freshly grated ginger

1 teaspoon olive oil

Half a teaspoon of cumin

½ teaspoon sea salt

Regarding the avocado-blueberry salsa

quarter cup of raw blueberries

1/4 cup of coarsely chopped red bell pepper or orange

1 tablespoon freshly chopped cilantro

One little avocado

METHODS TO BEGIN

- Put fish into a small plate. Mix the lime juice, cumin, ginger oil, and salt in a bowl. Use half of the lime mixture for the fish and save the remaining portion for the avocado-blueberry salsa. Turn fish to coat; let marinate at room temperature for 15 minutes.
- On medium-high heat, gently butter a grill pan. Fish should be drained and moved from the marinade to the grill pan. Remove the marinade from the dish. Fish should be cooked for 4 to 6 minutes

per 1/2 inch of thickness, or until it just starts to flake with a fork.

- To make the salsa, put the blueberries, cilantro, pepper, and saved lime mixture in a small bowl. Cut avocado into tiny pieces, then carefully mix it into the salsa. Up to four hours before serving, cover and refrigerate. Before serving, spoon the salsa over the swordfish.

25. Ahi Tuna Seared with a Ginger-Scallion Sauce

NUTRITION: 271 mg of sodium, 12 g of fat (2 g saturated), and 301 calories

4 SERVES
You'll need
1 bunch of roughly cut onions with their bottoms removed
Two tablespoons of freshly grated and peeled ginger
One teaspoon of low-sodium soy sauce
Three tablespoons of peanut oil
One tablespoon of rice vinegar

16 oz. premium tuna steaks, such as Ahi
Add pepper and salt to taste.
1½ pounds sliced shiitake mushrooms with stems removed
Baby bok choy, 1 pound, stems removed

METHODS TO BEGIN

- In a mixing bowl, add the scallions, ginger, soy sauce, vinegar, and 2 tablespoons of oil; toss to fully blend. Put away. (Preparing this in advance and putting it in the fridge is not only feasible but also advised, as the flavors will meld beautifully after even 30 minutes.)
- In a large cast-iron skillet or sauté pan, heat the remaining oil.
- Give the tuna a generous amount of salt and black pepper.
- Add the tuna to the pan and sear it for 2 minutes on each side, or until it is thoroughly browned, once the oil is just beginning to smoke. Delete.
- Add the shiitake mushrooms to the same heated skillet (if the pan becomes dry, add another dab of oil) while the tuna is resting. Add the bok choy and cook for

another 2 to 3 minutes, until gently browned. Sauté the bok choy for a further two to three minutes, or until it begins to soften. Use salt and pepper to season to taste.

- Cut the tuna into large, thick pieces. Arrange the mushrooms and bok choy on four heated plates.
- Place tuna pieces on top and pour the ginger-scallion sauce over them.

26.   Mahi-Mahi Grilled with Salsa Verde

NUTRITION: 390 mg of sodium, 15 g of fat (2.5 g saturated), and 280 calories

4 SERVES
You'll need
1/4 cup of freshly chopped parsley
1/4 cup of freshly chopped mint (optional)
lime juice from one
one-quarter cup olive oil (plus more for grilling)

Three chopped anchovy fillets; two tablespoons of rinsed and chopped capers; two finely minced garlic cloves
A dash of red chili powder
To taste, add salt and black pepper.
Four mahi-mahi fillets, or around 6 ounces of other firm white fish such as swordfish, halibut, or sea bass

METHODS TO BEGIN
- Warm up a grill. Ensure that the grate has been greased and cleaned.
- In a mixing bowl, combine the parsley, olive oil, lemon juice, capers, anchovies, garlic, and pepper flakes. If using, add mint.
- Use black pepper to season.
- Put the green salsa aside.
- After lightly oiling the fish, sprinkle salt and pepper on it all over.
- Lay the fillets skin side down on the grill and cook for 5 minutes, or until the skin peels away easily and is crisp and lightly browned (if you tamper with the fish before it's ready to flip, it will probably cling).

- When the salmon flakes with a light touch from your fingertip, turn it over and continue cooking for another two to three minutes on the other side.
- Spoon the salsa verde over the fillets before serving.

Suck This Advice
How to Get the Skin of Fish Crisp
All too often, we remove the skin off fish fillets and throw it away, missing out on one of the fish's healthiest and most delicious sections. When cooked to perfection, the skin adds a tactile contrast to the tender meat of the fish.

When cooking skin-on fillets, either on a grill or in a hot pan, cook the fillets for about three-quarters of the cooking time on the skin side before flipping them over and finishing on the flesh side.

Not every fish has skin designed to be crisp. Although the skin of swordfish, tilapia, and salmon is delicious, the skin of halibut, tilapia, and mahi-mahi should be thrown away, either before or after cooking.

Meats: Pig, Lamb, And Beef.

Beef Dishes

1. Plagiarised Big Mac Recipe

NUTRITION: 380 calories, 760 mg of sodium, and 15 g of fat (5 g saturated).

SERVES 4 ARE NEEDED
Two tablespoons of olive oil mayo
One tablespoon mustard
One tablespoon of ketchup
1 tablespoon grated onion
One tablespoon of sweet pickle relish
One tablespoon of Worcestershire sauce
One pound of sirloin
To taste, add salt and black pepper.
Cuts of four American cheeses

8 slices of dill pickles
½ cup finely chopped yellow onion
Four buns with sesame seeds gently toasted
One cup of iceberg lettuce, shredded

METHODS TO BEGIN

- In order to create the unique sauce, mix together the mayonnaise, mustard, ketchup, relish, chopped onion, and Worcestershire in a mixing dish.
- Shape the meat into eight equal balls.
- On a chopping board, press the balls into thin patties using your hands or a spatula.
- A big cast-iron skillet should be preheated to medium-high heat.
- Black pepper and salt should be used to season the patties on both sides.
- Add 4 of the patties to the pan once it's really hot.
- Cook for one minute or so, or until a brown crust forms.
- After flipping the patties, place a piece of cheese on top of two of them, and cook for an additional 60 to 90 seconds, or until the bottoms are crusty as well.

- Add two pickles and a handful of chopped onion on the top of each cheeseburger.
- After arranging the nude patties on the cheeseburgers, transfer them to a chopping board.
- Continue with the other four patties.
- Drizzle a liberal quantity of special sauce over the bottoms of the buns, then top with shredded lettuce.
- After placing the burgers on the buns and covering them with the bread tops, serve.

2. Plagiarized Taco Bell Cheese and Chili Burrito

Ingredients: 6 servings at a time
One-pound ground beef
One tablespoon of taco spice
Ten-ounce can of refried beans
One 6-oz tomato paste can
Relishable taco cheese
Six flour tortilla shells

METHODS TO BEGIN

- Heat a frying pan over medium heat.
- Grind the meat until it's no longer pink. Empty the surplus oil into a container.
- Add a dash of taco seasoning.
- Add the tomato paste and the cans of refried beans. Mix well to blend.
- Before assembling the tortilla, let the cheese and chili mixture warm up.
- To assemble the burrito, fill a tortilla shell with a portion of the chili cheese mixture and an equal quantity of cheese. Fold the tortilla in half.
- To press the tortilla, preheat another skillet. Once the bottom of the tortilla is toasted, add it to it and let it set for one to three minutes. Using a spatula to push down, flip the sandwich and toast the other side.
- Serve with leftover Taco Bell sauce packets, if you have them, or your favorite spicy sauce!

3. Meat Tacos

INGREDIENTS FOR 4 SERVINGS MADE
1 pound of beef ground
Taco seasoning, two teaspoons
Hard taco shells and half a cup of water
cheese tacos
lettuce with shredded pico de gallo

METHODS TO BEGIN
- According to the directions on the package, preheat the oven for the taco shells.
- While cooking the ground beef, pour off any extra fat into a can. It is harmful for your sink to spill fat down the drain.
- Mix the water with two teaspoons of taco seasoning. Simmer until the meat is well-composed and the sauce has thickened.
- The hard shell tortillas should be warmed in the oven.
- Arrange the taco meat, pico de gallo, shredded lettuce, and taco cheese on warmed shells.

4. Recipe for Slow Cooked Beef Goulash

NUTRITION: 12 g fat (5 g saturated), 12 g sugar, 9 g fiber, 559 mg sodium, and 378 calories.

Ingredients: 6 servings at a time
90% lean ground beef, one pound
Eight ounces of dry multigrain, high-protein elbow macaroni (2 1/3 cups) and 21/2 cups of reduced-sodium beef broth
One 15-oz can of tomato sauce without additional salt
One 14.5-oz can of chopped tomatoes without added salt
One 6-oz can of tomato paste without additional salt
1/2 cup of onion, chopped finely
half a cup of carrot shreds
Half a cup of coarsely chopped sweet pepper, green
1/4 tsp black pepper and 1/2 tsp salt
Half a cup of cheddar cheese, shredded

METHODS TO BEGIN

- Together with the pepper, mix the first 11 ingredients (in a 5- to 6-quart slow cooker). To crumble the ground beef, stir. Cook for two hours on high with a cover on, stirring once throughout the cooking process.
- Add a little cheese. Once the pasta is soft and the cheese has melted, simmer it covered for a further 10 minutes.
- Suck This Advice
- Generally speaking, one part protein, one part carbohydrate, and two parts non-starchy veggies should make up your supper plate. Serve this dish over greens!

5. Bowls of Beef Burritos

4 BOWLS' WORTH Ingredients
Four tablespoons of olive oil and one big head of cauliflower
Halal salt
Pepper, black

One big yellow onion and three bell peppers, thinly sliced
Two cups of halved cherry tomatoes
One-pound ground beef
1/4 tsp cumin
1/4 tsp paprika smoked
Two plump avocados
One little red onion cut finely
1 lime's juice

METHODS TO BEGIN

- Take off the cauliflower's core and stem, then cut or grate it finely to make it rice-like in texture.
- Fill a big pan with 2 tablespoons of olive oil and place it over medium-high heat. Add the cauliflower, 1/4 tsp salt, and 1/4 tsp pepper once the oil begins to shimmer. Cook for 5 to 8 minutes, stirring often, or until the cauliflower starts to soften.
- After the cauliflower is cooked, transfer it to a dish and clean the pan.
- In the skillet, add 1 tablespoon of olive oil and increase the heat to medium-high.

Add the onions, peppers, and 1/4 teaspoon of salt. Cook for approximately 5 minutes, stirring periodically, or until softened. After that, move the veggies to a platter. Avoid wiping the pan clean.

- The ground beef, cumin, paprika, and 1/2 tsp salt should all be added to the pan along with the remaining 1 Tbsp olive oil. Cook the beef over medium-high heat, breaking it up as necessary, until it is well-cooked and browned.
- Mash the avocados, red onion, and lime juice in a small bowl. To taste, add salt and pepper for seasoning.
- Spoon the ground beef, sautéed veggies, and cauliflower rice into four dishes. Serve with a generous dollop of guacamole on top.

6. Zingy skewers of teriyaki meat

Nutrition: each portion
NutrientUnit kcal 9g protein, 6g fiber, 46g carbohydrates, 22g saturates, and 563 fat
Salt (39g) 1.4g

Components

1 tablespoon soy sauce or tamari

3 tbsp orange juice, just extracted

15g of peeled and extremely finely grated chunk ginger and 2 crushed garlic cloves

One teaspoon of honey, ideally raw

1 tsp of chili powder

300g of tough-to-chew beef sirloin steak, sliced into long, thin strips

100g long-grain brown rice for the salad

One cucumber, sliced into little cubes

Using a peeler, peel and cut into ribbons two medium carrots

4 spring onions, cut into diagonal pieces and trimmed

100g of sliced and trimmed radishes

20g of coarsely chopped coriander leaves + more for garnish

10g of mint leaves, plus more for decoration

1 tablespoon juice and zest of cold-pressed rapeseed oil One lime

25g of unsalted cashew nuts, coarsely chopped and roasted

Procedure:

Step 1: In a small saucepan with 100ml cold water, combine the tamari, orange juice, ginger, garlic, honey, and chili flakes. Bring to a boil. Boil vigorously for 3 to 5 minutes, or until the mixture is well reduced, glossy, and slightly syrupy. Take off the heat, transfer it to a shallow dish, and allow it to cool.

STEP 2: Thread 4 wet skewers, either metal or wood, with the beef. After adding the marinade, turn it over and brush it well to coat. After 30 minutes of marinating, cover with cling film.

The recipe follows the advertisement below.

Step 3: Make the salad while the beef marinates. Pour half the water into a medium pan and heat it until it boils. Cook the rice according to the package directions for about 20 minutes or until it's tender. After rinsing in a sieve with cold running water, thoroughly drain. Pour into a large basin.

STEP 4: Combine the oil, lime zest and juice, cucumber, carrots, spring onions, radishes, coriander, and mint. Toss thoroughly. Add a pinch of black pepper for seasoning. Split between two dishes, then sprinkle some more herbs and almonds on top for decoration.

Step 5: Turn the grill's heat to high. (Alternatively, you could sear the skewers in a nonstick griddle pan.) Setting aside any extra marinade, place the skewers on a rack above a baking dish covered with foil. Cook the kebabs near the flame for three to five minutes on each side, or until cooked to your preference. When they are rotated, brush with additional marinade. When cooked, they should have a shiny, sticky appearance. Serve the rice salad hot or cold.

Lamb Dishes

1. Recipe for Lamb and Potato Cakes

This recipe yields 4 servings.
Prepare in 25 minutes.
Cook for ten minutes.
193 calories per serving

Ingredients: 250g sweet potato, 80g spring onions, and 25g fresh coriander leaves.
One clove of garlic
227g minced lamb
tsp allspice
Tomato puree, 16g
One tablespoon of Worcestershire sauce
20g of flour

Approach
- Boil sweet potatoes in diced form for ten to fifteen minutes, then remove and mash.
- Chop the coriander finely.

- Add the lamb and cook it gently for around five minutes, flipping it over regularly, in a nonstick pan until the onions and garlic are soft. Then, drain off any extra grease.
- Cook for two minutes, stirring regularly, after adding the potato, allspice, tomato puree, Worcestershire sauce, half of the chopped coriander, and salt and pepper to taste.
- Form the batter into eight 1-centimeter-thick cakes and dust with flour.
- Cakes should be dry-fried for two minutes on each side, or barbecued.
- Add the remaining coriander as a garnish.

Nutritional Data For Each Dish
Calories (193 kcal)
Protein (g) 12.0 Carbohydrate (g) 17.4 Fat (g) 8.9 Fiber (g) 2.0 Alcohol (g)   0.0 Fruit and Vegetable 1.1

2. Recipe for Lamb Stuffed Onions

This recipe yields 4 servings.
Ten minutes for prep
Cook for 40 minutes.
 196 calories per serving

Ingredients:
400g raw onions, average 168g lamb mince, average 0g ground cinnamon, average 0g powdered allspice
0g Whole Cumin Seeds Average 168 grams of raw spinach, average 2 thin slices of 60 grams of white, medium-sliced bread, average ¼ teaspoon of salt (1.25 grams), average ¼ teaspoon of freshly ground black pepper (0.5 grams), Standard 6g Beef Cubes, Stock Assist Weight, Whole, raw, 48-gram Oxo 1 small egg, weight with shell

Approach:
Step 1: Set the oven's temperature to 190°C (375°F, Gas Mark 5).
2. To make breadcrumbs, put the bread in a food processor and blitz.

3. After peeling the onions and cutting off the top and root ends to make them stand straight, hollow out the onion with a melon baller until the shell is 1 centimeter thick. Save roughly 225g of the onion seeds, then finely chop and set aside.

4. After submerging the onions in boiling water for around five minutes, remove them and place them upside down on a rack to drain.

5. Brown the lamb over medium heat and then drain any excess fat. Cook the onion until it becomes soft by adding the chopped onion and seasonings.

6. Include the spinach in the lamb mixture and cook it until it wilts. Then, take it off the heat and toss in the egg, breadcrumbs, and salt and pepper to taste.

7. Fill the onion shells with the lamb mixture after arranging them on an oven dish.

8. Fill the dish with stock, bake for 30 minutes, then cover and bake for an additional 10 minutes.

Nutritional Data For Each Dish
Energy (kcal)   196%
Protein (g) 13.0 Carbohydrate (g) 16.6 Fat (g) 8.6 Fiber (g)   2.5 Gum Alcohol   0.0 Fruit and Vegetable 1.9

3. Recipe for Masala Lamb Kebabs

This recipe yields 4 servings.
 fifteen minutes for prep
Cook for 25 minutes.
154 calories per serving

Components:
 2g of ground ginger
Stale coriander leaves, 5 grams
12.5g/½ teaspoon cinnamon
1/2 tsp cumin seeds
1 Tsp/4g of chili powder
5g masala garam
3g/1 Tsp turmeric

Lemon Juice (30ml)
Ten milliliters (two teaspoons) of sunflower oil
5g/1 Tsp salt
400-gram lamb chop

Approach

- Set oven temperature to 200°C (Gas Mark 6) or 400°F.
- In a large bowl, mix all the spices, oil, lemon juice, and salt.
- Tear the lamb into small pieces and combine it with the spice mixture.
- Allow the marinade to sit at room temperature for one hour, or refrigerate for at least three hours or overnight.
- Arrange the lamb chunks on skewers and place them on a baking sheet that has been gently oiled.
- Bake for 20 to 25 minutes, or until well cooked.
- Halfway through the cooking period, flip the skewers.
- Serve with a veggie curry and rice or naan bread.

Nutritional Data For Each Dish
154 calories (kcal)
Alcohol (g) 0.0 Fruit & Veg 0.1 Carbohydrate
(g) 2.9 Fat (g) 6.7 Protein (g) 20.9 Fiber (g) 0.4

4. Recipe for Lamb Stew

Makings for 6 servings
fifteen minutes for prep
Cook for 50 minutes.
221 calories per serving

Ingredients: 454g potatoes, 454g carrots, 180g
onion, and 454g lean lamb
One clove of garlic
White flour (20g)
20g cubes of lamb stock include
½ teaspoon dried thyme ½ gram dried bay
leaves

Approach
- Slice and peel the onion.
- Cut the carrots and potatoes into
  bite-sized pieces after peeling them.

- Chop and remove excess fat from the lamb.
- Garlic should be peeled and crushed before being added to a heavy-based skillet with chopped lamb. Brown over medium heat, rotating often.
- After covering the lamb with flour, fry it for one minute while stirring continuously.
- Prepare the stock and pour it into the pan, swirling to mix in any flour that may have clung to the pan.
- Add the potatoes, onions, and carrots; stir frequently and bring to a boil.
- Once the gravy has thickened, stir in the thyme and bay leaf, cover, and simmer until the meat and potatoes are very soft about 30 minutes.
- Accompany with freshly cooked veggies. If you're preparing for one person, just reheat leftovers from the freezer for a healthy, fast supper!

Nutritional Data For Each Dish
Calories (221 kcal)
Protein (g) 18.0 Carbohydrate (g) 22.5 Fat (g) 6.8 Fiber (g) 3.1 Glassware (g) 0.0 Fruit and Vegetable 1.4

5. Delicious Recipe for Lamb Hotpot

This recipe yields 4 servings.
Twenty minutes for prep
Cooking time: 1 hour; serving size: 368 calories

Components:
2 onions
Potatoes 700g, 4 carrots
2 teaspoons gravy granules
400g of lamb leg, lean
Two tsp finely chopped fresh mint
A spoonful of olive oil
1 cube of stock

Approach
- Set oven temperature to 325°F / Gas Mark 3 / 160°C.

- After slicing and peeling the potatoes, submerge them in cold water. Chop the onion and carrots, then cut the lamb into pieces.
- In a heavy pan, heat the oil, add the lamb, and cook it for ten minutes, or until it becomes brow.
- Extract pan juices and set aside. Toss in the carrots and onions with the meat. Add 5 minutes more to fry.
- Place the stock cube in and crumble in 350ml of hot water. Take the pan off of the burner and add the gravy granules.
- After moving the lamb to an oven-safe dish, cover it with potato pieces, drizzle with the fluids that were set aside, and season it well.
- For 40 minutes, bake. Garnish with chopped mint and serve.

Nutritional Data For Each Dish
Energy (kcal)   368)
Protein (g): 25.3 Fiber (g) Carbohydrate (g): 42.6 Fat (g): 11.2   Alcohol (g): 5.5   0.0 Fruit and Vegetable 2.2

6. Recipe for Grilled Lamb Chops

This recipe yields 4 servings.
35 minutes for prep
Cook for 20 minutes.
311 calories per serving

Components
Greek yogurt with 60g of low-fat
15g of dry mint
¼ teaspoon salt and ¼ teaspoon freshly ground pepper
500g chops of lamb

Approach
- Set the grill's temperature to medium.
- Add a tablespoon of dried mint to the Greek yogurt and season with salt and pepper. Cover the lamb chops with the mixture and let them marinate for half an hour.
- Grill for 8–10 minutes, rotating once, or until well cooked.
- Accompany with a fresh green salad.

Nutritional Data For Each Dish
Calories (311 kcal)
Protein (g) 27.5 Carbohydrate (g) 3.0 Fat (g)
21.0

Swine Recipes

1. Pork Chile Verde

NUTRITION: 460 calories, 620 mg of sodium,
24 g of fat (8 g saturated),

6 SERVES
You'll need
Tbsp canola oil
Cubes of pork shoulder, 2 pounds, boneless,
chopped to 1 inch
To taste, add salt and black pepper.
One cup of chicken broth with minimal sodium
One 15-oz bottle of salsa verde (Salsa verde is a
mild salsa composed of onions and tart
tomatillos. It goes well with eggs and tacos.)

1/4 of a medium onion

One large green bell pepper, cut into large pieces

Two cups of optional little fingerling or marble potatoes

8 tortillas de maiz

Cut two limes into quarters.

METHODS TO BEGIN

- In a large skillet or sauté pan, heat the oil over high heat.
- Use salt and pepper to season the meat.
- Pork should be added to the pan in stages and seared until it is caramelized on the surface but still uncooked on the inside. If the pork is packed too tightly, it will steam rather than brown.
- Put in a slow cooker after that.
- Pour the broth into the heated pan and scrape off any tasty, crispy pig pieces with a wooden spoon.
- Cover the pork with the broth, bell pepper, onion, and salsa verde.
- Once the pork is very soft, turn the slow cooker to high and simmer for 4 hours (or low for 8). Add the potatoes to the

saucepan during the last hour of cooking if you want to use them.

- Together with the stewed vegetables and a ladle of the cooking liquid, serve the pork in bowls.
- For impromptu tacos, have warm corn tortillas and lime chunks on hand.

2. Smothered Chops of Pork

NUTRITION: 15 g fat (6 g saturated), 720 mg salt, and 260 calories

4 SERVES
You'll need
Four center-cut, thick, bone-in pork chops, approximately 6 ounces each
To taste, add salt and black pepper.
Chopped cayenne
One tablespoon of butter
F2 tablespoons
One cup of chicken stock reduced in sodium
1/ cup buttermilk with less fat
1 teaspoon Dijon mustard
fresh parsley that has been chopped (optional)

METHODS TO BEGIN

- Season the chops with salt, black pepper, and a little amount of cayenne one hour before cooking, then put them back in the fridge. (You may omit this step, but doing so guarantees a chop that is more completely seasoned and juicy.)
- In a large cast-iron skillet or sauté pan, melt the butter over medium heat.
- Shake off any excess flour after gently dusting both sides of the chops with flour.
- Sear the chops for 4 minutes on each side, turning once, until well browned but not done through.
- Transfer to a chopping board.
- When the liquid has reduced by half, add the mustard, buttermilk, and stock to the pan and simmer for 5 to 7 minutes.
- After adding the chops back to the pan, simmer them for a further three minutes or so, or until they are cooked through.
- Pour the gravy over the chops before serving, and if desired, sprinkle some parsley on top.

3. Slow-Cooked Shoulder of Pork

NUTRITION: 900 mg of salt, 22 g of fat (8 g saturated), and 410 calories

SERVES 12 TO 16
You'll need
One (6–8 lb) Without bones pork shoulder
two tsp salt
1/4 cup of sugar, granulated
A half-cup of brown sugar

METHODS TO BEGIN
- Rub the pork all over with the granulated sugar and salt the night before cooking. To let the brine sit overnight, cover it and put it back in the fridge.
- Set oven temperature to 300°F.
- Transfer the pork to a sizable baking dish and cook it on the lower rack. Baste the pig about every 30 minutes using a big spoon or baster. (If you want, the pork may be left in the oven without basting, and it will still turn out delicious.)

- The pork is done after approximately five hours, or when a fork can easily pierce it.
- After taking the pork out of the oven, raise the temperature to 475°F.
- After giving the pork a thorough coat of brown sugar, put it back in the oven.
- Roast until a rich mahogany crust develops on the sugar, approximately 15 minutes.
- Serve either as is or in any of the ways described in "Meal Multiplier," below, with a few veggie sides.

4. Sautéed Apples with Teriyaki Pork Chops

NUTRITION: 890 mg of sodium, 9 g of fat (3.5 g saturated), and 315 calories

4 SERVES
You'll need
Four 6-ounce pork chops apiece
One cup of teriyaki marinade (such as Soy Vay) in a bottle
1/2 tablespoon canola or peanut oil
½ chopped onion

1 teaspoon freshly grated ginger
One apple, chopped, peeled, and cored
a half-cup of apple juice
1/4 cup vinegar made from apples
1 teaspoon powdered Chinese five-spice
To taste, add salt and black pepper.

METHODS TO BEGIN

- In a shallow dish or sealable plastic bag, combine the pork chops and teriyaki sauce, flipping the chops to coat.
- Refrigerate the bowl or bag to allow it to marinade for at least one hour and up to eight hours.
- Heat up a big cast-iron skillet, grill pan, or barbecue.
- Heat the oil in a medium saucepan over medium heat while the grill preheats.
- Cook the onion and ginger together for around two minutes, or until the onion becomes transparent.
- Stir together the apple, vinegar, five-spice, and apple juice.
- Reduce the heat and let it simmer for around ten minutes, or until the fruit is tender but not mushy and the liquid has

enough thickened to somewhat cling to the apples.

- After preheating the grill or pan, take the pork out of the marinade, using paper towels to remove any excess, and cook it for 4 to 5 minutes on each side, or until it is firm but gives slightly when touched. The marinade's sugars can burn if the grill is too hot, so proceed with caution. The ideal temperature is a pleasant middle one.)
- Spoon a little of the apple chutney over each chop.

5. Low-Calorie Sandwich with Pulled Pork

CALORIES: 430, FAT: 18 g (5 g saturated), SOD: 540 mg

12 SERVES
You'll need
One 4-to 5-pound boneless pork shoulder
To taste, add salt and black pepper.
½ tablespoons vegetable or canola oil
Apple cider vinegar, one cup

Four cups of chicken broth reduced in sodium
1½ tablespoon liquid smoke
12 hamburger buns (Martin's Potato Rolls work well)
Coleslaw recipe

METHODS TO BEGIN
- A big skillet or sauté pan should be heated to medium-high heat.
- Slice the pork into two or three large chunks, then sprinkle with salt and pepper.
- When the oil is heated, add it to the pan and sear the pork chunks until the exterior is well browned. After removing the meat, put it in a slow cooker.
- When the pan is heated, add the vinegar and deglaze it, being sure to scrape off any browned meat residue on the bottom.
- Cover the pig with the vinegar, then cover again with the broth and liquid smoke.
- After turning the slow cooker on to high, simmer the pork for 4 hours, or until it easily crumbles under light pressure.
- After taking the pork out of the liquid, shred it. Serve with coleslaw on top of

heated buns after tossing with a little additional vinegar.

6. Roast Pork Loin in the Style of Porchetta with Lemony White Beans

nutriTION: 350 calories, 410 mg of sodium, and 10 g of fat (3 g saturated).

4 SERVES
You'll need
three minced garlic cloves
grated orange zest from two
Spoonful of fennel seeds
1 1⁄2 tablespoons freshly chopped rosemary
tsp olive oil
One 2-pound pork loin, ideally still with a little bit of fat around it
To taste, add salt and black pepper.
Two 16-ounce cans each Rinse and drain cannellini, Great Northern, or white kidney beans.
lime juice from one

METHODS TO BEGIN

- Set oven temperature to 450°F.
- Garlic, orange zest, fennel seeds, and 1 tablespoon of rosemary should all be combined on a chopping board.
- Make several passes with your knife through the mixture until it starts to resemble paste. Transfer it to a bowl and drizzle with the olive oil.
- After adding salt and pepper for seasoning, massage the mixture all over the meat.
- You may now cook it right away or, for a more flavorful result, marinade the loin in the fridge for up to 4 hours.
- Depending on the thickness of the loin, place the pork in a roasting pan and roast it for 25 to 30 minutes, or until an instant-read thermometer put into the center registers 150° to 155°F.
- Take out of the oven and give it a 10-minute rest before slicing.
- Mix the beans, lemon juice, and the remaining ½ tablespoon of rosemary in a saucepan and heat until the ingredients

are well warmed, while the pork is resting.

- Add pepper and salt for seasoning. Arrange the pork pieces on top of the beans.

7. Lean Pork Chops Dredged in Balsamic Honey Dressing

nutriTION: 340 mg of sodium, 19 g of fat (9 g saturated), and 300 calories

4 SERVES
You'll need
one-fourth cup balsamic vinegar
Two tablespoons of butter
two tsp honey
1 tsp freshly chopped rosemary
1/four teaspoon red pepper flakes
Four well-sliced pork chops
To taste, add salt and black pepper.

METHODS TO BEGIN
- In a small saucepan over medium heat, cook the balsamic vinegar, butter, honey,

rosemary, and pepper flakes until the butter melts and the mixture starts to bubble gently. Take off the heat source.

- Set a grill or grill pan to preheat.
- About 2 teaspoons of the balsamic glaze should be transferred to a small bowl and left there. After liberally seasoning the pork chops with salt and pepper, drizzle them with the leftover glaze.
- Depending on thickness, cook the pork for 3 to 4 minutes on each side after the grill reaches a medium-hot temperature. (A thermometer put into the thickest section of the chop should register 140°F for excellent medium pork.)
- After removing the chops, brush them with the reserved glaze using a clean brush.

8. Pineapple salsa paired with grilled pork tenderloin

NUTRITION: 390 mg of sodium, 4 g of fat (1.5 g saturated), and 210 calories
SERVES 4 ARE NEEDED

1 tablespoon grainy mustard (Dijon)
1/2 teaspoon honey
A half-tsp of chili powder
To taste, add salt and black pepper.
1/4-inch-thick pineapple slices with the core removed and one pound of pork tenderloin
One red onion, chopped
One minced jalapeño pepper
1/2 cup of freshly chopped cilantro
1 lime's juice

METHODS TO BEGIN

- Warm up the grill.
- Rub the pork all over with a mixture of mustard, honey, chili powder, and a generous pinch of salt and pepper.
- Arrange the pineapple pieces and meat on the grill.
- The pineapple should be softened and faintly browned after 2 to 3 minutes on each side of the grill.
- The tenderloin should be lightly browned and firm to the touch, with an internal thermometer reading no higher than 160°F, after approximately 10 minutes of grilling, rotating the meat once or twice.

- Give the pork at least five minutes to rest.
- Dice the pineapple into small pieces while the pork is resting.
- Mix in the lime juice, cilantro, onion, and jalapeño.
- Add a little salt and pepper for seasoning. After slicing, serve the pork with the salsa.

9. Grilled pork chops with peaches, both sweet and savory

NUTRITION: 24 g fat (8 g saturated), 530 mg salt, and 430 calories

TWO SERVES
You'll need
Four bone-in, thick-cut (1") pork chops (8 oz each); prepackaged chops are sliced too thinly, which makes them dry out quickly. To ensure that they retain moisture and taste during cooking, ask the butcher to cut them thick and on the bone.
Olive oil.

To taste, add salt and black pepper.
Two hard peaches or nectarines, cut in half and with pits
Two tablespoons of toasted pine nuts and one little red onion, cut thinly
1/2 cup of blue cheese, crumbled
One tablespoon balsamic vinegar

METHODS TO BEGIN

- Turn a grill to high heat.
- After seasoning with salt and pepper, drizzle the pork with olive oil.
- Grill each side for 4 to 5 minutes.
- The flesh should be bright pink in the center, but the exterior should be scorched rather than burnt.
- Brush the peach halves with oil and place them on the grill, cut side down, while the chops are cooking.
- Grill until soft, about 5 minutes. Take it out, cut it into slices, and combine it with the vinegar, blue cheese, onion, and pine nuts. Add salt and pepper to taste.
- Place half of the peach mixture on top of each chop before serving.
-

10. Savage Jerk Pork

NUTRITION: 510 mg of sodium, 11 g of fat (2 g saturated), and 240 calories

4 SERVES
You'll need
Two habanero or Scotch bonnet peppers, stemmed and coarsely diced (Note: To handle the peppers, either wear gloves or minimize skin contact by using tongs.)
Approximately 8 scallions, chopped
Lime juice from two
2 tablespoons canola oil
three chopped garlic cloves
tsp allspice
1½ teaspoon nutmeg
To taste, add salt and black pepper.
Pork loin, 1 pound

METHODS TO BEGIN

- In a food processor, combine the habaneros, scallions, lime juice, oil, garlic, allspice, nutmeg, and a generous amount of salt and pepper.
- Add a little amount of water if the mixture seems too dry and pulse until it forms a paste the consistency of pesto.
- Pour the jerk marinade over the pork (chicken drumsticks also work very well) in a plastic bag that can be sealed.
- To ensure that the pork is covered evenly, release any remaining air, close the bag, and give it a few rubs.
- Let the food marinate for a minimum of one hour, ideally overnight.
- Warm up a grill.
- After removing the pork from the marinade, add a little extra salt and pepper to taste.
- Grill for approximately ten minutes, turning occasionally, or until cooked through and lightly browned on both sides. (An internal thermometer placed in the pork's middle will register 140°F.)

Candy With A Small Amount Of Bite

Recipe 1: Yogurt Fruit Parfait

Ingredients:
1 cup non-fat Greek yogurt
1 cup mixed fresh fruits (such as berries, diced apples, or sliced bananas)
2 tablespoons honey or agave syrup
1/4 cup granola or crushed nuts (optional)

Procedure:
In a glass or small bowl, layer the yogurt and mixed fruits.
Drizzle honey or agave syrup over the fruit and yogurt.
Top with granola or crushed nuts for added texture and flavor.

Preparation Time:
Preparation time is approximately 5-10 minutes.

Nutritional Information:

Calories: 150
Total Fat: 0.5g
Saturated Fat: 0g
Cholesterol: 5mg
Sodium: 35mg
Total Carbohydrates: 30g
Dietary Fiber: 2g
Sugars: 20g
Protein: 10g

Recipe 2: Vegetable and Hummus Snack

Ingredients:
Assorted sliced vegetables (such as cucumbers, carrots, and bell peppers)
1/2 cup hummus

 Procedure:
Arrange the sliced vegetables on a plate.
Serve with hummus for dipping.

Preparation Time:
Preparation time is approximately 5-10 minutes.

Nutritional Information:
Calories: 100
Total Fat: 5g
Saturated Fat: 1g
Cholesterol: 0mg
Sodium: 150mg
Total Carbohydrates: 12g
Dietary Fiber: 5g
Sugars: 3g
Protein: 4g

Recipe 3: Baked Apple Chips

Ingredients:
2-3 apples, thinly sliced
Cinnamon to taste

Procedure:
Preheat the oven to 200°F (95°C).
Place the thinly sliced apples on a baking sheet lined with parchment paper.
Sprinkle cinnamon over the apple slices.
Bake for 1.5 to 2 hours until the chips are crispy.

Let cool before serving.
 Preparation Time:
Preparation time is approximately 10 minutes.
Baking time is 1.5 to 2 hours.

Nutritional Information:
Calories: 50
Total Fat: 0g
Saturated Fat: 0g
Cholesterol: 0mg
Sodium: 0mg
Total Carbohydrates: 14g
Dietary Fiber: 2g
Sugars: 10g
Protein: 0g

Recipe 4: Tuna and Avocado Lettuce Wraps

Ingredients:
1 can of tuna, drained
1 ripe avocado, mashed
Salt and pepper to taste
Lettuce leaves

Procedure:
In a bowl, mix the drained tuna and mashed avocado.
Season with salt and pepper.
Scoop the mixture onto lettuce leaves and wrap.

Preparation Time:
Preparation time is approximately 10-15 minutes.

Nutritional Information:
Calories: 200
Total Fat: 10g
Saturated Fat: 1.5g
Cholesterol: 30mg
Sodium: 250mg
Total Carbohydrates: 10g
Dietary Fiber: 6g
Sugars: 1g
Protein: 20g

Recipe 5: Cucumber and Cottage Cheese Bites

Ingredients:
1 medium cucumber, sliced
1/2 cup low-fat cottage cheese
Fresh dill or chives for garnish

Procedure:
Place a dollop of cottage cheese on each cucumber slice.
Garnish with fresh dill or chives.

Preparation Time:
Preparation time is approximately 5-10 minutes.

Nutritional Information:
Calories: 80
Total Fat: 2g
Saturated Fat: 1g
Cholesterol: 10mg
Sodium: 250mg
Total Carbohydrates: 6g
Dietary Fiber: 1g
Sugars: 4g

Protein: 8g
Recipe 6: Whole Grain Pita and Hummus

Ingredients:
1 whole grain pita, cut into triangles
1/4 cup hummus

Procedure:
Toast the whole grain pita until crisp.
Serve with hummus for dipping.

Preparation Time:
Preparation time is approximately 5-7 minutes.

Nutritional Information:
Calories: 150
Total Fat: 3g
Saturated Fat: 0g
Cholesterol: 0mg
Sodium: 200mg
Total Carbohydrates: 26g
Dietary Fiber: 5g
Sugars: 1g
Protein: 6g

Recipe 7: Banana Oatmeal Cookies

Ingredients:
2 ripe bananas, mashed
1 cup rolled oats
1/4 cup chopped nuts or seeds (optional)
1/4 teaspoon cinnamon

Procedure:
Preheat the oven to 350°F (175°C) and line a baking sheet with parchment paper.
In a bowl, mix the mashed bananas, rolled oats, chopped nuts or seeds, and cinnamon.
Drop spoonfuls of the mixture onto the baking sheet.
Bake for 12-15 minutes until golden brown.

Preparation Time:
Preparation time is approximately 10-15 minutes. Baking time is 12-15 minutes.

Nutritional Information:
Calories: 100
Total Fat: 3g
Saturated Fat: 0.5g

Cholesterol: 0mg
Sodium: 5mg
Total Carbohydrates: 17g
Dietary Fiber: 2g
Sugars: 6g
Protein: 3g

Recipe 8: Baked Sweet Potato Fries

Ingredients:
2 medium sweet potatoes, cut into strips
1 tablespoon olive oil
Salt and pepper to taste

Procedure:
Preheat the oven to 425°F (220°C) and line a baking sheet with parchment paper.
Toss the sweet potato strips with olive oil, salt, and pepper.
Arrange the strips on the baking sheet in a single layer.
Bake for 20-25 minutes, flipping halfway through.

Preparation Time:
Preparation time is approximately 10 minutes.
Baking time is 20-25 minutes.

Nutritional Information:
Calories: 120
Total Fat: 3g
Saturated Fat: 0.5g
Cholesterol: 0mg
Sodium: 200mg
Total Carbohydrates: 22g
Dietary Fiber: 3g
Sugars: 5g
Protein: 2g

Recipe 9: Zucchini Pizza Bites

Ingredients:
2 medium zucchinis, sliced into rounds
1/2 cup marinara sauce
1/2 cup shredded mozzarella cheese
Italian seasoning to taste

Procedure:
Preheat the oven to 400°F (200°C) and line a baking sheet with parchment paper.
Place the zucchini rounds on the baking sheet.
Top each round with marinara sauce and shredded mozzarella cheese.
Sprinkle Italian seasoning over the bites.
Bake for 10-12 minutes until the cheese is bubbly and golden.

Preparation Time:
Preparation time is approximately 15-20 minutes. Baking time is 10-12 minutes.

Nutritional Information:
Calories: 80
Total Fat: 3.5g
Saturated Fat: 2g
Cholesterol: 10mg
Sodium: 150mg
Total Carbohydrates: 8g
Dietary Fiber: 2g
Sugars: 4g
Protein: 5g

Recipe 10: Oatmeal Banana Muffins

Ingredients:
2 ripe bananas, mashed
1 cup rolled oats
1/4 cup honey or maple syrup
1/4 cup Greek yogurt
1 teaspoon baking powder

Procedure:
Preheat the oven to 350°F (175°C) and line a muffin tin with paper liners.
In a bowl, mix the mashed bananas, rolled oats, honey or maple syrup, Greek yogurt, and baking powder until combined.
Divide the mixture evenly among the muffin cups.
Bake for 15-20 minutes or until a toothpick inserted in the center comes out clean.

Preparation Time:
Preparation time is approximately 10-15 minutes. Baking time is 15-20 minutes.

Nutritional Information:
Calories: 120
Total Fat: 2g
Saturated Fat: 0.5g
Cholesterol: 5mg
Sodium: 100mg
Total Carbohydrates: 25g
Dietary Fiber: 3g
Sugars: 12g
Protein: 3g

Soups And Other Beverages

1. Bacon and Chicken Orzo Soup

Prepare in ten minutes.
Take 35 minutes to cook
Forty-five minutes total
Six servings
281 calories

INGREDIENTS Metric; US Customary
Five bacon slices
Two cups of chopped yellow onions (about one big onion)
two minced garlic cloves
One cup of chopped celery (about three ribs)
one cup chopped carrots
One-pound chicken breast, skinless and boneless
Six cups of homemade, preferably chicken stock
half-cup pasta
One and a half tsp kosher salt, or to taste
One-half teaspoon of freshly ground black pepper, or to taste, finely chopped fresh parsley

DIRECTIONS

- Render the bacon grease over low heat in a large Dutch oven or heavy-bottomed saucepan. After the pan has a beautiful coating of fat on the bottom, increase the heat a little bit and fry the bacon until it becomes crisp. To drain, place the bacon on a platter covered with paper towels. Save no more than two to three tablespoons of the grease in the pan.

- Toss in the carrots, celery, onions, and garlic, and season with salt. The more caramelization you get from the veggies, the more delicious the final soup will be. Cook the vegetables over medium heat for a few minutes, stirring them from time to time.

- Place the chicken breasts over the veggies and pour the chicken stock over them. After bringing the liquid to a boil, turn down the heat and cover. Simmer the soup for twenty minutes. After removing, transfer the chicken to a chopping board.

After the meat has cooled down a little, shred it with two forks. Put away.

- Add the orzo and return the soup to a boil. Cook, uncovered until the orzo is al dente, about 8 minutes.

- Reintroduce the chicken to the broth and adjust the seasoning with salt and pepper.

- Chop the bacon you set aside. Before serving, top each bowl of soup with chopped bacon and fresh parsley. (Note: You may reheat bacon in the microwave for 10-second bursts or in a pan over medium heat.)

2. Hot Sausage, Whole-Wheat Orecchiette Soup with Kale

Components
Two tsp of olive oil
One chopped sweet onion and 1/4 teaspoon of salt
One-fourth tsp black pepper

Crushed red pepper flakes, 1/2 teaspoon
4 minced garlic cloves
Six cups of chicken stock (low sodium)
One pound of hot Italian turkey sausage
One cup of whole wheat macaroni
Four cups of fresh kale cut into pieces after removing the stems
Add extra grated Parmigiano Reggiano cheese for dusting; 1/4 cup fresh

DIRECTIONS

- Add the olive oil to a big saucepan that is heated over medium-low heat. Stir in the onion after adding the salt, pepper, and red pepper flakes. Stirring regularly, cook until onions soften, approximately 5 minutes. After adding the garlic and cooking it for a further minute, raise the heat to medium-high and boil the liquid. Next, add the chicken stock.
- Preheat a large nonstick pan over medium-high heat while the stock is heating. If the sausage is in a casing, take it out and add it to the pan along with a dash of salt and pepper. Using a wooden spoon, split the sausage into smaller

pieces (or any desired size) while it cooks for 6 to 8 minutes, or until it is browned. Cut the heat off.

- Pasta should be added to the boiling stock and cooked for 8 to 10 minutes or until al dente. Stir well and simmer for a further two minutes after adding the greens. Add the cheese, taste, and adjust the seasoning with more salt and pepper to taste. You may either pour the whole sausage into the soup or portion it out into bowls and top each one with a slice of sausage. Present with more cheese for slicing. To avoid the noodles becoming too mushy, be sure to turn off the heat under the soup.

3. Lime and Jalapeño Chicken Soup

Components
Two tsp of olive oil
Diced half a red onion, minced two jalapeños (ribs and seeds removed), and four cups water
One tsp salt (add more if necessary)

One pound of skinless, boneless chicken thighs
or breasts
Two 14-oz cans of drained white beans
(cannellini or Great Northern)
One sixteen-ounce jar of salsa verde made with
fresh cilantro from two limes, sour cream, and
cheese shreds for serving

DIRECTIONS

- Saute the onion and jalapeño in olive oil
  in a soup pot over medium heat until they
  become tender and aromatic.
- Mix in the salt and water. Heat till
  boiling. Chuck in the chicken breasts,
  raw. Cook for five to ten minutes with a
  lid on. Take off the heat, but don't take
  the cover off so the chicken cooks for a
  further 20 minutes. Take out and place
  the chicken breasts aside to cool.
- To the saucepan, add the salsa and white
  beans. Simmer over medium heat for half
  an hour.
- Return the chicken to the pot after
  shredding it.
- Pour the juice of one lime into the
  saucepan just before serving. To serve,

cut the remaining lime into wedges. Salt is added; taste and adjust as necessary. Accompany with shredded cheese, sour cream, and fresh cilantro.

NOTES: After Step 2, save the liquid and strain the mixture through a fine screen to eliminate any undesirable chicken fat from the broth. Bring the liquid back to a medium boil in the pot. To get rid of any chicken fat, you may also just scrape over the surface.

- This is great eaten on its own or as a side dish with white rice. It lessens the heat somewhat.
- Instant Pot: Add chicken, beans, salsa verde, red onion, water, salt, and jalapeños to the Instant Pot. Cook on the soup setting for 10 minutes, then quickly release the pressure. Shred the chicken and add one lime juice to the soup. Accompany with shredded cheese, sour cream, and fresh cilantro.

4. Egg Drop Soup with Bacon

Components

Chicken broth, 4 cups

two minced garlic cloves

Two chopped scallions stalks

1 1/2 tsp freshly grated ginger

1/4 teaspoon on the ground

Six strips of bacon, prepared and sliced into 1-inch pieces (I use turkey, but any sort would do).
To taste, soy sauce
Red chili powder, for flavor

1-tsp black pepper

two tsp cornstarch

three eggs

Approach

- Add the first 8 ingredients to a large saucepan over medium-high heat, along with 1/2 teaspoon of black pepper. After bringing it to a boil, lower the heat to a simmer. Simmer for 20 minutes with a lid on.
- Combine the cornstarch and two tablespoons of broth in a small bowl. Put away.

- Beat eggs with the remaining half teaspoon of black pepper in a separate bowl. Pour into the soup gradually while stirring. then gradually whisk in the cornstarch mixture after that.
- After tasting to adjust the spices, dig in!

5. Corned beef and cabbage soup prepared slowly

Components
4 tsp poultry stock

One 12-ounce bottle of beer (pale ale was my choice)

1.5 pounds of large-chunk corned beef

1.5 pounds of bite-sized chopped Yukon gold potatoes

Two chopped and peeled carrots

two celery stalks, chopped

One medium-sized white onion, chopped and peeled

One small head of chopped, cored, and shredded green cabbage

a large teaspoon of salt, freshly ground black pepper, and one bay leaf

fresh parsley, chopped, to serve.

DIRECTIONS

- In a large slow cooker bowl, add all ingredients and stir to mix. Once the beef is soft and readily shreds, simmer it covered for 7-8 hours on low or 3–4 hours on high.
- Take the chunks of beef out of the stew and shred it into bite-sized pieces with two forks. Stir the steak back into the stew once it has been removed. After

tasting and adding more salt and pepper
if necessary, take off the bay leaf.
- If preferred, top warm servings with
  freshly chopped parsley.

6. Asian Chicken Noodle Soup with Spices

Components:
1 tsp olive oil
One medium onion, diced (about half a cup)
One medium carrot cut into half-circles and
sliced (approximately 1/2 cup sliced)
Five big cloves of garlic, finely chopped
(approximately five tablespoons)
One tsp carefully shredded fresh ginger root
Thinly slice two fresh Thai chilies (omit the
seeds for a milder kick).
Four ounces of freshly sliced neatly stemmed
shiitake mushrooms
4 cups chicken stock reduced in sodium
A pair of filtered glasses
Two one-pound, skinless, boneless chicken
breasts

6 ounces, or half a bag Extra Broad Noodles by No Yolks®
Two to three teaspoons of dark soy sauce, or as a garnish, chopped fresh cilantro to taste

Instructions:

- Place a large pot or Dutch oven over medium heat and add the olive oil. Add the onion and carrot and sauté for 3 to 4 minutes, or until the onion and carrot are somewhat softened. Next, add the mushrooms and cook for an additional 3 minutes, or until the mushrooms are tender and have decreased in size. Stir in the garlic, ginger, and chilies for about a minute, or until fragrant.
- Simmer after adding the water and chicken broth. When the thickest section of the chicken reaches 165 degrees Fahrenheit on an instant-read thermometer, the chicken is cooked through, so add the chicken breasts to the broth and simmer for 10 to 15 minutes. Take the chicken out of the saucepan and place it on a platter to cool down a little before using a fork to shred it.

- To the boiling broth mixture, add the noodles and cook for 7 to 8 minutes, or until they are just al dente. Return the shredded chicken to the saucepan and heat it for an additional one to two minutes. Add soy sauce and stir to taste.
- Distribute among serving dishes and sprinkle chopped cilantro on top.

Beverages

1.   Ginger-Lemon Detox Water:

Ingredients:
1 inch of fresh ginger, thinly sliced
1 lemon, thinly sliced
4 cups of water

Procedure:
Combine ginger and lemon slices in a pitcher.
Pour water over the mixture and refrigerate for
2-4 hours.
Serve over ice.

Preparation time: 5 minutes (plus 2-4 hours for
chilling)

2. Berry and Spinach Smoothie:

Ingredients:
1 cup fresh spinach
1 cup mixed berries (strawberries, blueberries,
raspberries)
1 cup low-fat yogurt
1 tablespoon honey (optional)

Procedure:
Blend spinach, berries, and yogurt until smooth.
Add honey if desired and blend again.

Preparation time: 5 minutes

3. Cucumber Mint Limeade:

Ingredients:
1 cucumber, sliced
1/4 cup fresh mint leaves
1 lime, juiced
4 cups of water
Ice cubes

Procedure:
Combine cucumber slices and mint in a pitcher.
Add lime juice and water, then stir well.
Serve over ice.

Preparation time: 10 minutes

4. Pineapple-Kale Green Juice:

Ingredients:
1 cup fresh pineapple chunks
2 cups kale leaves
1 cucumber, sliced
1/2 cup water

Procedure:
Juice pineapple, kale, and cucumber.
Add water to dilute as needed.
Preparation time: 5 minutes

5. Turmeric Almond Milk:

Ingredients:
2 cups almond milk
1 teaspoon turmeric
1/2 teaspoon cinnamon
1 teaspoon honey (optional)

Procedure:
Heat almond milk in a saucepan.
Add turmeric and cinnamon, and stir until well
combined.
Sweeten with honey if desired.

Preparation time: 5 minutes

6. Minty Watermelon Refresher:

Ingredients:
2 cups watermelon, cubed
1/4 cup fresh mint leaves
2 cups water
Ice cubes

Procedure:
Blend watermelon and mint with water until smooth.
Serve over ice.

Preparation time: 5 minutes

7. Carrot and Orange Juice:

Ingredients:
4 medium carrots, chopped
2 oranges, peeled and segmented

Procedure:
Juice carrots and oranges together.
Stir well before serving.

Preparation time: 5 minutes

8. Coconut Water Smoothie:

Ingredients:
1 cup coconut water
1 banana
1/2 cup pineapple chunks
1/2 cup spinach

Procedure:
Blend all ingredients until smooth.
Serve chilled.

Preparation time: 5 minutes

9. Beetroot and Apple Juice:

Ingredients:
1 medium beetroot, peeled and chopped
2 apples, cored and chopped

Procedure:
Juice the beetroot and apples together.
Stir well and serve immediately.

Preparation time: 5 minutes

10. Mixed Berry Iced Tea:

Ingredients:
2 black tea bags
1 cup mixed berries (strawberries, blueberries, raspberries)
4 cups water
Ice cubes

Procedure:
Steep tea bags in hot water for 5 minutes.
Add mixed berries and let cool.
Serve over ice.

Preparation time: 10 minutes

11. Cinnamon Apple Smoothie

Ingredients:
1 apple, cored and chopped
1 cup low-fat yogurt
1/2 teaspoon cinnamon

1 tablespoon honey (optional)

Procedure:
Blend apple, yogurt, and cinnamon until smooth.
Sweeten with honey if desired.

Preparation time: 5 minutes

12. Tomato and Basil Mocktail:

Ingredients:
2 tomatoes, chopped
1/4 cup fresh basil leaves
1/2 teaspoon black pepper
1/2 teaspoon salt
2 cups water

Procedure:
Blend tomatoes and basil with water until smooth.
Season with black pepper and salt.
Serve chilled.

Preparation time: 10 minutes

13. Mango and Avocado Smoothie:

Ingredients:
1 ripe mango, peeled and chopped
1/2 ripe avocado, peeled and chopped
1 cup low-fat milk
1 tablespoon honey (optional)

Procedure:
Blend mango, avocado, and milk until creamy.
Sweeten with honey if desired.

Preparation time: 5 minutes

14. Pomegranate and Blueberry Juice:

Ingredients:
1 cup pomegranate seeds
1 cup blueberries
1 cup water

Procedure:
Blend pomegranate seeds and blueberries with
water until smooth.
Strain the juice if desired.

Preparation time: 5 minutes

15. Lemon-Basil Iced Tea:

Ingredients:
2 black tea bags
1/4 cup fresh basil leaves
1 lemon, sliced
4 cups water
Ice cubes

Procedure:
Steep tea bags and basil in hot water for 5 minutes.
Add lemon slices and let cool.
Serve over ice.

Preparation time: 10 minutes